i

BIOETHICS
IN REAL LIFE

www.ingramcontent.com/pod-product-compliance
Lightning Source LLC
Chambersburg PA
CBHW050506210326
41521CB00011B/2344

THE CENTER FOR

BIOETHICS
& HUMAN DIGNITY

TRINITY INTERNATIONAL UNIVERSITY

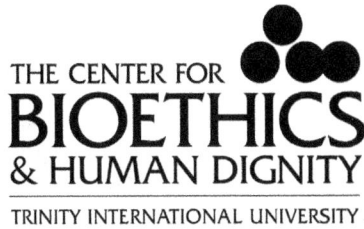

The Center for Bioethics & Human Dignity (CBHD) is a Christian bioethics research center at Trinity International University that explores the nexus of biomedicine, biotechnology, and our common humanity. CBHD fosters a distinctly Christian conception of bioethics that is both academically rigorous and broadly accessible. From within a Judeo-Christian Hippocratic framework, we anticipate, interpret, and engage the pressing bioethical issues of our day. As a center of rigorous research, theological and conceptual analysis, charitable critique, and thoughtful engagement, we bring clarity to the complex issues of our day.

Our Origins:

In 1993, more than a dozen leading Christian bioethicists gathered to assess the noticeable lack of explicit Christian engagement in the crucial bioethics arena. This group sponsored a major conference in May 1994, "The Christian Stake in Bioethics," and concurrently launched The Center for Bioethics & Human Dignity. In 2007, CBHD formally became a center of Trinity International University.

Our Involvement:

Over the years, the Center has initiated a variety of projects, including a number of conferences, consultations, and publications. As a leading voice, CBHD staff and fellows have appeared in a wide range of print, radio, and television news sources. In addition, the Center has collaborated over the years with a variety of organizations, including the Christian Medical and Dental Associations, Nurses Christian Fellowship, and the Christian Legal Society, as well as international institutions including the Centre for Bioethics and Public Policy and the Linacre Center both in London, England, the Lindeboom

THE CENTER FOR
BIOETHICS
& HUMAN DIGNITY
TRINITY INTERNATIONAL UNIVERSITY

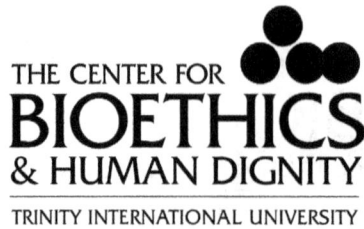

BIOETHICS IN REAL LIFE:
LESSONS WE'RE LEARNING FROM COVID-19

Edited by
Dónal P. O'Mathúna, Bryan A. Just, Wilson Jeremiah,
and F. Matthew Eppinette

Layout and Design Editing by Catherine Klug & Curtis Wayne Pierce, Jr.

The Center for Bioethics and Human Dignity
Deerfield, Illinois

Published 2022 by The Center for Bioethics & Human Dignity
2065 Half Day Road
Deerfield, IL 60015

Print: 978-1-7357653-0-3
Ebook: 978-1-7357653-1-0
PDF: 978-1-7357653-2-7

Suggested citation:
Dónal P. O'Mathúna, Bryan A. Just, Wilson Jeremiah, and F. Matthew Eppinette, eds. *Bioethics in Real Life: Lessons We're Learning from COVID-19* (Deerfield, IL: The Center for Bioethics & Human Dignity, 2022).

www.cbhd.org

CONTENTS

EDITORS' INTRODUCTION

DÓNAL P. O'MATHÚNA, PHD

BRYAN A. JUST, MA

WILSON JEREMIAH, THM

F. MATTHEW EPPINETTE, MBA, PHD

The chapters in this book are all adapted from presentations given at CBHD's 27th annual summer conference, *Bioethics in Real Life: Lessons We're Learning from COVID-19*. Held in June 2020, *Bioethics in Real Life* was most certainly not the conference we expected to hold that year, nor did we expect to offer an entirely online conference. Nevertheless, we are thankful we were able to connect virtually for the conference, even if it was an unexpected development.

As a point of reference, recall what the early days of the COVID-19 pandemic were like in the United States. On April 15, 2020, a YouTuber who goes by the moniker "Microsoft Sam" uploaded a "video supercut" entitled "Every COVID-19 Commercial Is Exactly the Same."[1] The video, which is about four minutes long and was viewed more than a million times in the first few weeks after it went live on YouTube, pokes fun at the way every company that produced a commercial addressing the pandemic seemed to be working from the same script. From the somber piano music that gradually builds throughout each scene to the generic camera shots, one could be forgiven for thinking that a single director was in charge of every commercial.

Even the scripts seem to have been copied from one another, as the video splices together dozens of companies rehashing phrases like "since [founding date of company]," "in these difficult/troubling/challenging/ trying/uncertain/unprecedented times," "people," "we're here for you," "now more than ever," "family," "together," and "home." The video ends with a montage of people applauding, with images from ads by Samsung, Google, and MasterCard reminding us of the practice of going outside to applaud healthcare workers each evening.

It is truly difficult to do justice in print to this video, so we encourage you to watch it for yourself. What you will see are brands large and small—global, national, regional, and local in reach—all using similar music, images, and words to advertise during the early weeks of the pandemic in the United States.

Many people took this "supercut" to be making fun of the companies and their ad agencies. Indeed, this seems to be Microsoft Sam's intent. In the video's description he writes:

> many companies have found themselves short on cash, almost overnight. They needed to get a message out—and quick. They asked their teams to throw something together. Since they can't film a new ad because of social distancing, they compiled old stock b-roll footage and found the most inoffensive, royalty-free piano track they could. This, combined with a decade of marketing trends dictated by focus groups and design-by-committee, released a tsunami of derivative, cliche ads all within a week of one another.[2]

Certainly, this is one way to understand these ads, and perhaps some of these criticisms are valid. However, if we take a step back, we might see that there is a bit more to these ads than lazy and clichéd self-promotion. Our suggestion is that there are so many common elements to the ads because there was a commonality about the experience those of us in the United States went through in the first weeks of the COVID-19 pandemic.

Yes, the music draws us in. Indeed, it is similar to the music we selected for the introduction video for the *Bioethics in Real Life* conference.[3] We all have a history, even companies and brands. The similarities in the commercials reflect the more serious similarities in many people's experiences. Many "people" have been left feeling isolated. We were, in many cases, separated from friends, loved ones, and "family." Many of us were at "home," "now, more than ever." These times were indeed "difficult," "troubled," "challenging," and "unprecedented." Our collective experience, particularly in the last two weeks of March and the first two weeks of April 2020, when these commercials were released, was filled with uncertainty.

We were, and in some ways remain, uncertain about what it is that we know and do not know. To borrow from a former Secretary of Defense, with some slight paraphrasing:

> there are known knowns . . . things we know that we know . . . there are known unknowns . . . some things we are aware of not knowing. But there are also unknown unknowns—things that we do not yet realize we are unaware of.[4]

During the early days of COVID-19, we were using the phrase "radical, dynamic uncertainty" to describe our situation. It was unlike any kind of uncertainty most of us had experienced, and it was happening globally. The information we were receiving was frequently shifting; it seemed as if every day some new or contradictory piece of information was presented or discovered, so that what was true one day was called into question the next. We were unsure how long this would last, what effect it would have on society, and even from whom we should receive our information. Over a year later, many of these questions remain unanswered, creating a common experience of radical, dynamic uncertainty. More questions have been added as we move through different surges in cases, grapple with policies about how best to shut down or re-open, and struggle with ethical considerations about how to allocate, globally distribute, or even mandate COVID-19 vaccines.

Notice, however, that we are sharing a common experience, not a universal experience. Indeed, while there has been much uncertainty, much else about the COVID-19 experience has varied greatly for different people. Within the field of healthcare, some have been pushed to the very edge of their limits, sometimes assigned to departments outside of their expertise and/or overwhelmed with caseload. Others in healthcare found themselves furloughed, their income cut, or stuck at home. As wave after wave of cases has come through our hospitals, some find themselves practicing while exhausted, some have left their beloved professions, and others have been fired for refusing to be vaccinated. Though this example is specific to healthcare, similar situations can be found across many professions. So, by way of orientation, recall that, particularly in the early weeks of the pandemic, we shared an experience with much in common, but it was not a universal experience.

The chapters in this book help us to unpack the common yet disparate experiences of the pandemic. They cover numerous topics related to COVID-19, including research, vulnerable populations, moral injury, resource allocation, and the value of human life. These, of course, are not all of the issues we might examine or the questions we might ask. But they are, we would like to suggest, a not insignificant sampling.

Perhaps fittingly for this shared experience, several themes arise in multiple chapters. Uncertainty is one of these—as Dónal O'Mathúna writes, "uncertainty abounds!" But this uncertainty does not have to be debilitating. Rather, it presses us to seek out the best information we can find within reasonable, carefully balanced standards. We have an obligation to learn. Uncertainty also reminds us to be discerning regarding the information we take in. Read carefully. Consider thoughtfully. Choose wisely.

Uncertainty, fear, isolation, and feelings of abandonment are all wrapped up together in the midst of the current pandemic. James Mc-Clendon beautifully describes the virtue and practice of presence as "being one's self for someone else . . . refusing the temptation to withdraw mentally and emotionally; but it is also on occasion putting our own body's weight and warmth alongside the neighbor, the friend, the lover in need."[5] The pandemic, for a time, put sharp limits on our ability to practice this virtue of presence. This is a genuine loss, one that must be acknowledged and grieved. We would do well to be mindful of the loss of presence in the lives of those around us, and indeed in our own lives.

The role of faith, of the biblical witness, and of the community of faith are emphasized by our authors in various ways. It is good to be reminded, and to have these brought to the forefront of our minds. Several authors will also mention the concept of solidarity: we are in this together (recall the commercial supercut). We are mutually bound to one another, and we need to both acknowledge and embrace our mutual dependence. Thus, we may carry and share the burdens of others. None of us stands on our own personally or professionally, nor should we think that we do. Solidarity means that empathy and love lead to action.

Empathy and love leading to action embodies the concept of neighbor-love, which Matthew Eppinette and Bryan Just discuss in the opening chapter. One way in which we might define neighbor-love is seeing the needs and interests of others as at least as important as our own needs and desires. They explore this further through the parable of the Good Samaritan, and its implications for the Christian stake in the current pandemic.

In his chapter, O'Mathúna looks at the ethics of research during a pandemic. Considering the unknowns and uncertainty that arose from a novel coronavirus, solid research is crucial. But it must also be ethical. He explores many of these ethical issues in research and the use of randomized controlled trials, using four case studies regarding research carried out in 2020 to show how these issues arose in very practical ways.

Joseph Wiinikka-Lydon's chapter focuses specifically on moral distress and moral injury. Moral distress can be both a healthy and a necessary response to traumas experienced in the healthcare setting! The circumstances in which distress and injury occur are influenced by multiple factors far beyond the immediate circumstance: public opinion, culture, and politics writ large. Acknowledging and confronting these factors can be both healing to those who have experienced this trauma and can serve as a catalyst for change.

COVID-19 has been a global pandemic, a reality that is well-recognized by Bramwel Wekesa. Writing from Kenya, his chapter considers the specific challenges faced in the African context. Many of these challenges will seem familiar to non-African readers, but others are unique, reminding us again that although there may be many common experiences of COVID-19, these are not necessarily universal.

For his chapter, Matthew Anderson approaches the issues of lockdowns and other governmental policies meant to curb the spread of SARS-CoV-2 through the lens of the *imago Dei*. He unpacks this Christian doctrine and its implications for the value we place on human life and the responsibilities we have to each other, as well as the ways that governments, hospitals, and individuals can use these insights in creating policy. He rejects both a strict "vitalism" that would require us to accept zero risks and a strict utilitarianism that values only the young and healthy, instead developing and applying a nuanced view of the value of human life.

Catherine Glenn-Foster addresses the importance of formulating laws and policies on fundamental ethical principles. Foremost amongst these, she argues, should be "a profound respect for human life as a gift of such inestimable worth that the loss of a single person diminishes every one of us." The COVID-19 pandemic has raised many ethical challenges, of which Glenn-Foster addresses four: the ethical allocation of scarce healthcare resources in patient care; ensuring that the elderly and those with disabilities are cared for with dignity, especially around visitation policies and end-of-life care; balancing pandemic response with the provision of routine medical care, including childbirth and surgery; and countering the pressures to promote abortion during the pandemic. Each of these ethical issues is challenging and highlights the importance of approaching all of them with a deep respect for human life.

One of the factors that exacerbated the COVID-19 pandemic was that very few were prepared for such a far-reaching event. Healthcare systems did not have space for the influx of patients or supplies to treat them. Worldwide supply chains were not prepared for the disruption of lockdowns. Government policy was outdated or ill-prepared for this kind of crisis. However, in his concluding chapter, Cheyn Onarecker points out that in addition to these areas, we were not prepared *ethically* for the COVID-19 pandemic. He focuses on three main principles—the duty to treat, respect for the dignity of all persons, and caring for the caregiver—and the ways in which COVID-19 forced societies to make ethical decisions in each of these areas. He contends that thinking through these issues is crucial to preparing ourselves for the next pandemic or crisis.

Given the amount of information appearing about COVID-19, and how quickly it appeared, some aspects of this volume would have been out-of-date even if it had been published the week after the conference. As editors, therefore, we asked the authors to keep their chapters largely as presented, rather than attempt to keep updating them during each phase of publication. While this has the effect of dating some of the information, we believe that the ethical arguments presented by the authors remain cogent and important.

Each of the writers brings clarity, precision, and nuance to the topic he or she addresses, which is so vitally important to the task of loving our neighbor. Our task is not to ask questions about who our neighbor is; our task is to love all who are in need, regardless of race, color, age, or stage of development. Each is a unique person deserving of our care. We can only truly love our neighbor when we understand well what his or her needs are and how we might best go about meeting those needs. We discover or uncover our neighbor's needs through personal engagement and by careful research that is accompanied by thoughtful, discerning evaluation. We love our neighbors more fully and more authentically as we better understand the context in which they and we live, as we meet them in the midst of their distress, and as we properly recognize their infinite value.

It is our hope that the present work will better equip you to love your neighbor truly and fully. This, of course, is not the final word on bioethics and COVID-19. Far from it. Even as we complete this manuscript, we find ourselves in the midst of yet another surge in cases and now facing "a pandemic of the unvaccinated."[6] Ongoing examination and reexamination of the topics addressed in this book—as well as others—will be required in order to navigate the current and future pandemics well. May God grant us grace, wisdom, and understanding as we proceed through these uncertain times—together.

Notes

1. Microsoft Sam, "Every COVID-19 Commercial Is Exactly the Same," YouTube, April 15, 2020, https://youtu.be/vM3J9jDoaTA.

2. Microsoft Sam, "Every COVID-19 Commercial Is Exactly the Same."

3. The Center for Bioethics & Human Dignity, "2020 Conference Opener—'Bioethics in Real Life: Lessons We're Learning from COVID-19,'" YouTube, June 26, 2020, https://youtu.be/qTrl1-4dl34.

4. Donald Rumsfeld, "DoD News Briefing—Secretary Rumsfeld and Gen. Myers," U.S. Department of defense, February 12, 2002, available via https://web.archive.org/web/20160406235718/http://archive.defense.gov/Transcripts/Transcript.aspx?TranscriptID=2636.

5. James William McClendon, Jr., *Ethics: Systematic Theology*, vol. 1, 2nd ed. (Nashville, TN: Abingdon Press, 2002), 116.

6. Rochelle Walensky, quoted in Emily Anthes and Alexandra E. Petri, "C.D.C. Director Warns of a 'Pandemic of the Unvaccinated,'" *The New York Times*, July 22, 2021, https://www.nytimes.com/2021/07/16/health/covid-delta-cdc-walensky.html.

BIOETHICS AND PANDEMIC: FRAMING THE DISCUSSION

F. MATTHEW EPPINETTE, MBA, PHD

BRYAN A. JUST, MA

One task of this chapter, which was developed from the introductory address at the *Bioethics in Real Life: Lessons We're Learning from COVID-19* conference, is to provide a sketch of the Christian stake in the topic under discussion. We could frame the Christian stake in the COVID-19 pandemic or any global health crisis in a number of different ways. However, this is a good opportunity to turn to a familiar story.

Luke tells us of a man who was going down from Jerusalem to Jericho. He was attacked, robbed, stripped, beaten, and left for dead. A priest happened upon the scene, but he passed by on the other side of the road. A Levite, too, saw the man and passed by on the other side.

But a Samaritan, as he traveled, came where the man was; and when he saw him, he took pity on him. He went to him and bandaged his wounds, pouring on oil and wine. Then he put the man on his own donkey, brought him to an inn and took care of him. The next day he took out two denarii and gave them to the innkeeper. "Look after him," he said, "and when I return, I will reimburse you for any extra expense you may have" (Luke 10:33–35, NIV).

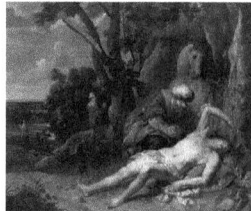

Around 1647, Flemish artists Balthasar van Cortbemde (1612–1663) painted a depiction of this familiar parable that, in a single image, captures a great deal of the story.[1] The Samaritan is seen in the foreground attending to the man, pouring what appears to be oil onto a wound on the right side of the man's chest. To the left, at some distance, the Levite is looking back over his shoulder, and in the far distance, almost at the edge of the frame, the priest walks on, reading a scroll as he goes.

A second painting, by Rembrandt (1606–1669), shows his interpretation of how the Samaritan at the inn might have appeared. Depicted in a setting more reminiscent of the Renaissance than the ancient near east, the Samaritan speaks with the innkeeper while someone helps the now bandaged man down off of the Samaritan' horse.[2] Cortbemde and Rembrandt tell almost the whole story in just two evocative, memory-triggering images.

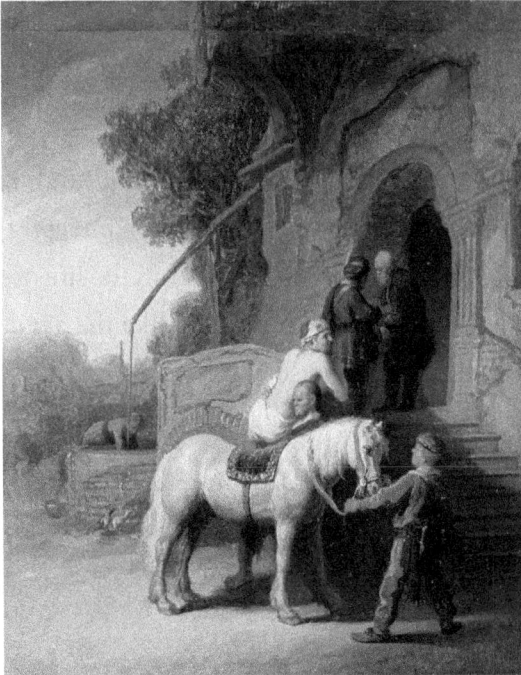

Of course, not only do we know the story, we know its context. An expert in the law is testing Jesus:

> "Teacher," he asked, "what must I do to inherit eternal life?"
> "What is written in the Law?" he replied. "How do you read it?"
> He answered, "'Love the Lord your God with all your heart and with all your soul and with all your strength and with all your mind'; and, 'Love your neighbor as yourself.'"
> "You have answered correctly," Jesus replied. "Do this and you will live."
> But he wanted to justify himself, so he asked Jesus, "And who is my neighbor?" (Luke 10:25b–29)

Luke concludes this account by revisiting the context once more:

> "Which of these three do you think was a neighbor to the man who fell into the hands of robbers?"
> The expert in the law replied, "The one who had mercy on him."
> Jesus told him, "Go and do likewise." (Luke 10:36–37)

It is easy to overinterpret this passage. Indeed, as Riemer Roukema details, the history of interpretation of this account holds several creative, allegorical readings.[3] It is also possible to under-interpret the episode; to see it as merely an interesting interaction from the life of Christ, with no bearing on us when it comes to something like the academic discipline of bioethics. But, in between these extremes, there is a way of allowing the text to speak to us today.

The direct and central point, of course, is "Which of these three do you think was a neighbor to the man who fell into the hands of robbers?" Or, in other words: Was it the priest, the Levite, or the Samaritan who actually loved this man?

The law expert's question seems to seek some limitation on who he might be called upon to love—recall that "he wanted to justify himself" (Luke 10:29). It is as if he were asking, "What are the parameters for, the limitations on, the boundaries of my neighborliness, of my love?" Jesus' parable inverts any expectation of limitations, however, pointing to the stranger, the unexpected one—we might even say to the least expected person—as our neighbor, as the one who is to be the recipient of our love. We might even go so far as to say that seeking limits on our neighborliness is the wrong approach entirely. Rather, we are to have an expansive view of neighbor and neighborhood. Our neighbor is anyone we encounter who has a need, and our neighborhood is wherever we find ourselves. We are to love those who need love no matter who they are or where they might be; to show the same mercy as the Samaritan.

The word the NIV renders as "mercy" could have been translated "compassion."[4] These are both familiar terms, and in some ways are closely related. Compassion, as we have all no doubt heard, carries the idea of suffering alongside another. Notice the action and activity of the Samaritan: he went, bandaged, poured, put, brought, and took care. This then was an active mercy, compassionate action.

Our suggestion is that active, compassionate care is at the very core of bioethics and even more so healthcare. Today, we have many controversies involving the issue of medical futility, or what is often (unfortunately) referred to as "futile care." This brings to mind something the late Dr. Bob Orr said regarding this term, which he strongly rejected, and rightly so: "Care is never futile. Treatment may be futile, but care is never ever futile." Bioethics rightly conceived is an activity of loving our neighbor rightly, properly, and actively.

Notably, rightly loving our neighbor is not something we do in isolation. Tom Cavanaugh draws attention to a character in the parable who is often overlooked: the innkeeper.[5] The innkeeper serves as a reminder of the cooperative nature of caring for others. It is not something that we do solely on our own, but in conjunction with others. Look again at Rembrandt's work, which includes not only the injured man, the Samaritan, and the innkeeper but also a man helping the injured man off the animal, someone tending to the animal, and someone else observing from a window. This scene demonstrates that the work of caring happens within a community of others who help and support not only the injured or sick person but also one another.[6]

When Matthew speaks to college and high school students about bioethics, he will often turn to this text because engaging in the work of bioethics involves both loving God and loving neighbor. We love God as we seek to be conformed to the image of Christ, as we seek to develop and live out Godly character, and as we seek to wisely apply Godly character to the dilemmas that arise in the context of life and health. This work engages the whole person: heart, soul, mind and strength.

The work of our conference, and the chapters in this book that flow from it, display the work of the mind, with implications for the work of the heart, the soul, and the strength of each of us. To those reading the proceedings of a Christian bioethics conference, it likely goes without saying that love of neighbor is clearly and directly relevant to the work of healthcare. Still, though, it is good to pause, remind ourselves of this, and reflect on the ways in which providing healthcare, participating in ethics consults, studying, writing, and speaking on the issues of bioethics involve love of neighbor.

Our point is simply this: in the midst of COVID-19, raising and examining questions and issues such as the ones we are raising and examining here are an important part of loving our neighbors both near and far. A conference like *Bioethics in Real Life: Lessons We're Learning from Covid-19* and a book like this also show the cooperative and communal nature of caring for others.

One of the other things one can take away from the story of the Good Samaritan—which most certainly is *not* the point of the story—is the fact that it provides a terrific example of a feature shared by almost all stories that have endured and been celebrated, namely, a three-act structure: introduction, complication, resolution. A story with a three-act structure first introduces us to a character or characters, places them in a context, and sets the action in motion. Soon, however, the character is beset by some complication with which he or she must struggle. Ultimately, though, a good and satisfying story resolves the complications.

The account of the Good Samaritan epitomizes this three-act structure:

- Introduction: A man went down from Jerusalem to Jericho.
- Complication: He was attacked, robbed, stripped, beaten, and left for dead.
- Resolution: A Samaritan bound up his wounds, carried him to safety, and saw to it that he was taken care of.

If it turns out that the story of COVID-19 has a three-act structure, we should keep in mind that we are still very much in the midst of the complication. While the story of the Good Samaritan is told with an economy of words, and much of the story can be portrayed in two paintings, this is not true of the story of COVID-19. Indeed, there is likely to be much more complication before we get to resolution in this story. Comparing headlines from the week of the conference to those of the following summer emphasizes this:

- Fox Carolina (June 25, 2020): "The 3 Most Populous States Are

Breaking Coronavirus Records"[7]

- CBS (June 24, 2020): "New Coronavirus Cases in U.S. Jump to Highest Level in 2 Months, Since Peak Of Outbreak"[8]
- *New York Times* (June 24, 2020): "Coronavirus Surge Raises Alarm as States Report New Highs"[9]
- *Associated Press* (July 23, 2021): "Edwards Calls for Return to Masks Indoors Amid COVID Spike"[10]
- *The Guardian* (August 3, 2021): "Covid Hospitalizations Rise across US as Hospitals Say Patients Aren't Vaccinated"[11]

Of course, the framework of loving God and loving neighbor does not in itself provide us with all of the answers for what we "should pursue and shouldn't pursue in matters of life and health."[12] But it does, we would like to suggest, provide us with an attitude or a posture that pushes us toward seeking to identify issues of significance in the midst of COVID-19, working to develop wise approaches to these issues, and considering ways in which we might go about putting that wisdom into place and practice. It also pushes us toward an iterative process of examining and reexamining our actions, attitudes, and priorities as this pandemic proceeds and then, we pray, recedes, and as we prepare for future crises.

Endnotes

1. This is a faithful photographic reproduction of a two-dimensional, public domain work of art. Faithful reproductions of two-dimensional public domain works of art are public domain. The original is in the Royal Museum of Fine Arts Antwerp. https://commons.wikimedia.org/wiki/File:Balthasar_van_Cortbemde_-_The_Good_Samaritan.jpg.

2. This work is in the public domain in its country of origin and other countries and areas where the copyright term is the author's life plus 100 years or fewer. https://upload.wikimedia.org/wikipedia/commons/f/f1/Rembrandt_Harmensz._van_Rijn_033.jpg.

3. Riemer Roukema, "The Good Samaritan in Ancient Christianity," *Vigiliae Christianae*, 58, no. 1 (2004): 56–74. As but one example, "Jerusalem stood for paradise and Jericho for the world into which man had fallen by the agency of the demons, whereas the Samaritan represented Christ" (57).

4. Walter Bauer, *A Greek-English Lexicon of the New Testament and Other Early Christian Literature*, rev. and ed. Frederick W. Danker, 3rd ed. (Chicago: University of Chicago Press, 2000).

5. Tom A. Cavanaugh, "Relating Hippocratic and Christian Medical Ethics," *Christian Bioethics*, 26, no. 1 (2020): 81–94.

6. The Duke University Health and Humanities Lab produced a brilliant and moving 14-minute documentary on the important roles played by hospital housekeeping and environmental services personnel. Entitled *Keepers of the House* and available on YouTube, this short film deserves a much wider audience: Duke Franklin Humanities Institute, *Keepers of the House*, YouTube, January 23, 2020, https://youtu.be/fNqMWNsm8wY.

7. Faith Karimi and Douglas Wood, "The 3 Most Populous States Are Breaking Coronavirus Records, Leading to Fears of 'Apocalyptic' Surges," Fox Carolina, June 25, 2020, https://www.foxcarolina.com/the-3-most-populous-states-are-breaking-coronavirus-records-leading-to-fears-of-apocalyptic-surges/article_649353ce-b257-5ab4-bfdf-8b79746d691e.html.

8. "New Coronavirus Cases in U.S. Jump to Highest Level in 2 Months, Since Peak of Outbreak," CBS News, June 24, 2020, https://www.cbsnews.com/news/coronavirus-cases-united-states-highest-peak/.

9. Matt Phillips and Anupreeta Das, "Coronavirus Surge Raises Alarm as States Report New Highs," *The New York Times*, June 24, 2020, https://www.nytimes.com/2020/06/24/business/stocks-markets-coronavirus.html.

10. Melinda Deslatte, "Edwards Calls for Return to Masks Indoors Amid COVID Spike," *Associated Press*, July 23, 2021, https://apnews.com/arti-

cle/health-coronavirus-pandemic-bec05dd9e2939c50b08a8b26fd0e8141.

11. Amanda Holpuch, "Covid Hospitalizations Rise across US as Hospitals Say Patients Aren't Vaccinated," *The Guardian*, August 3, 2021, https://www.theguardian.com/us-news/2021/aug/03/us-covid-coronavirus-cases-hospitalizations-unvaccinated.

12. John F. Kilner and C. Ben Mitchell, *Does God Need our Help? Cloning, Assisted Suicide, and Other Challenges in Bioethics* (Wheaton, IL: Tyndale House,

RESEARCH TO THE RESCUE? GENERATING EVIDENCE ETHICALLY FOR COVID-19

DÓNAL P. O'MATHÚNA

Overview

The chapter will examine the role of research during the COVID-19 pandemic, particularly the related ethical issues. First, I will examine some issues around research methods, particularly whether randomized controlled trials (RCTs) are necessary or ethical during COVID-19. This will lead into discussion about research ethics itself, where I will develop the view that research ethics needs to address more than just the ethical approval process and institutional review boards (IRBs), and address ethical issues that surround and encompass the whole research process. Four cases related to COVID-19 research will be examined, discussing ethical issues arising with three pharmaceuticals proposed for COVID-19 and then COVID-19 vaccines. The chapter will conclude with some suggestions about ways that biblical wisdom can help address these ethical issues.

Introduction

The COVID-19 pandemic can be characterized by uncertainty. As Gordon et al. stated early in the pandemic, "There are no antiviral drugs with proven clinical efficacy, nor are there any vaccines that prevent infection with SARS-CoV-2, and efforts to develop drugs and vaccine are hampered by the limited knowledge of the molecular details of how SARS-CoV-2 infects cells."[1] More generally, "We currently know little about what constitutes a protective immune response against COVID-19."[2]

Even with all this uncertainty, decisions must be made by clinicians, patients, and policy-makers. Research plays an important role in providing some of the missing information. Research can thereby contribute to the pandemic response. Without the evidence that research can provide, decisions will be made in the dark. As a result, people can be harmed from using ineffective interventions and delays in identifying effective responses. This leads to an ethical imperative to conduct research in the midst of the uncertainty. The World Health Organization (WHO) concluded that "conducting research is linked to 'a moral obligation to learn as much as possible, as quickly as possible.'"[3] In so doing, "research—implemented as policy and practice—can save lives."[4] This can reduce the harm from the pandemic, and help move things closer to something more normal sooner rather than later.

This moral obligation should lead to research being integrated into the pandemic response from the beginning. We cannot wait until the acute crisis passes to initiate research. Research is needed to help provide evidence to guide all phases of the response. At the same time, research has to be prioritized. Every evidence gap cannot be addressed immediately. Resources and personnel for research are limited and must be balanced against other needs, especially taking care of patients. A prioritization process should be established that must itself be conducted ethically. This includes ensuring that the needs of those directly impacted by the pandemic, both as patients and responders, are identified and addressed.

As needs are identified, various research questions will be generated. These questions can be addressed by different research methodologies. For example, determining whether a pharmaceutical is effective in treating COVID-19 requires a different methodology compared to understanding the lived experiences of those with COVID-19. Given the urgency of identifying effective treatments for COVID-19, research into such interventions should be high on any priority list. This has raised ethical questions about the best type of study design. In normal circumstances, randomized controlled trials are the established method for demonstrating efficacy. However, during a crisis, some have questioned whether these are appropriate.

Kim et al. have stated that "In critical situations, large randomized controlled trials are not always feasible or ethical, and critically ill patients may need to be treated empirically during times of uncertainty."[5] They conclude that small sample sizes, unvalidated end points, non-random allocation procedures, and unblinded studies "may be acceptable." They and others hold that during a crisis, when people are dying from a serious and novel disease, randomly and blindedly allocating participants to different groups is unethical, especially if some patients will receive a placebo (or sugar pill). The image is presented that some patients will be abandoned to receive no care in a placebo group, while others will receive a potentially effective treatment. What this image fails to acknowledge is that the experimental intervention could harm patients. Part of the purpose of research is to figure out whether an experimental intervention helps or harms. Being experimental does not guarantee benefit. At the same time, the comparison or control group can receive all of the standard care they would receive, just not receive the experimental intervention. They could end up benefiting from being in this group if the experimental intervention turns out to have adverse effects. Hence, RCTs are key to finding out if an intervention is effective or not, although there can be situations when they might not be feasible or ethical. The cases discussed later will show that an RCT can be conducted during a pandemic, and therefore should be used to address questions of efficacy.

This does not mean that RCTs are the only research methods need-ed. Qualitative and quantitative studies are required to provide differ-ent types of evidence needed in public health crises.[6] When addressing whether an intervention is effective, or if one is more effective than an-other, RCTs are the best study design. When other study methods are used to support questions of effectiveness, uncertainty continues and harm can result, as the cases below will demonstrate. Conducting RCTs during a pandemic is challenging but can be done. Methodological and ethical rigor must be maintained, especially when evidence is needed urgently. "But with speed borne of desperation comes risk and confu-sion—of trials too small to yield answers, of treatments overhyped, and of uncertainty about how to design the best studies possible."[7] Without rigorous studies, the results can be meaningless or incorrect. Effective interventions may be dismissed or ineffective interventions promoted, prolonging patient suffering and wasting resources and time. Uncertain-ty and confusion will continue to reign and may even undermine public trust in research and the scientific process.

Balance is needed. If we are overly cautious, clinical development will be hindered or delayed, and patients will be left without treatments for longer. If we are insufficiently cautious, patients will be exposed to un-known risks, and resources will be drained by ineffective interventions. "In both cases, misestimation threatens the integrity of the scientific en-terprise, because it frustrates prudent allocation of research resources."[8]

The way forward is not to reduce rigor or to cut corners, but to find ways to get the best possible research done. Adjustments may be needed, such as changing how projects are funded or receive ethical approval. Flexibility may be needed, but not in ways that undermine the rigor or ethics of the study. "We have to do our best science to make sure that we answer the questions as definitively as possible."[9] Only then will the world get the answers that it needs.

London and Kimmelman have proposed five recommendations for research that will guide our discussion of four cases.[10] First, studies should address important evidence gaps, which means that research studies will have to be prioritized. This should include ethical considerations, since those impact how priorities are determined. Second, rigorous designs are required to provide the best evidence for patients, clinicians and health systems. Questions of effectiveness and efficacy—whether one intervention works better than another—require RCTs. Questions around people's experiences require qualitative methods, such as interviews or focus groups. Third, trial designs should be prespecified, registered, and analyzed according to their protocols. It is human nature to be drawn towards what we think is best, and protocols (prespecified plans for research studies) provide a practical mechanism to counteract those biases in conducting research. Fourth, reports should be published promptly, completely, and consistent with the prespecified analyses in the protocols. Fifth, trials should be feasible so that they can recruit enough participants and finish on time. This includes ensuring that all relevant groups and populations are included as participants. We are already seeing concerns that African Americans are underrepresented in research studies, even though they make up a large proportion of the COVID-19 patient population in the US.[11]

Research Ethics

Before proceeding to the cases, a few comments are needed on research ethics. In addressing the ethical issues with COVID-19 intervention research, a broader approach to research ethics will be taken than one focused on ethics approval and IRBs. Research with human participants must be reviewed by committees which evaluate the ethical issues and can issue approvals for projects to begin. While such approval procedures are important, they can become the main or sole focus of research ethics. However, a growing consensus holds that ethics approval should be seen as only one element of research ethics, otherwise some ethical issues will not receive the attention they deserve.[12] For example, decisions are made during the design of trials that have ethical dimensions, such as which participants will be included. Engaging with the communities in which research will be conducted, and allowing them to have a voice in what topics are researched, is increasingly seen as ethically appropriate if not required.[13] Such decisions raise important ethical issues and are addressed before the study goes to an IRB. Likewise, when the results of studies are disseminated, ethical commitments are involved to ensure that researchers report results accurately and with appropriate restraint. Others, such as sponsors and the media, should also present the results accurately. In addition, clinicians and patients have ethical responsibilities as they use research evidence in their decision-making.[14] For example, clinicians should critically appraise the studies they read or hear about, not jumping to conclusions because they support previously held beliefs or biases.

All stakeholders in the research enterprise, from funders to researchers to consumers of evidence, have ethical responsibilities. And throughout the research process, not just during the IRB application process, ethical considerations must be taken into account. This requires a broad approach to what is viewed as research ethics. We will look at examples of these sorts of ethical issues as we examine the following four cases.

Case 1: Ivermectin

Ivermectin has been on the market for about 30 years. It is FDA-approved for oral use in treating parasitic worms and topical use for head lice and rosacea. Billions of doses have been distributed for use in animals and humans, with an excellent safety record.[15]

Interest in ivermectin for COVID-19 was sparked by a report on April 3, 2020 entitled "The FDA-Approved Drug Ivermectin Inhibits the Replication of SARS-CoV-2 *in vitro*."[16] The last two words are very important, meaning that the study was not carried out in animals but in laboratory containers. Public interest was fueled by media reports which often did not provide crucial details from the scientific report. For example, a report in *Newsweek* discussed the lab-based results, but not the doses involved.[17]

The original study noted that at 10 times the FDA-approved dose, ivermectin was *not* effective at killing the COVID-19 virus. Others calculated that the FDA-approved dose of ivermectin for humans would be 50 to 100 times lower than that required to kill the virus.[18] While the lab results are interesting, the high doses that would be required mean that these results are far from showing that this drug can be used safely or effectively. Other lab research has shown that ivermectin can inhibit RNA viruses, such as the viruses that cause dengue, Zika, and yellow fever. The COVID-19 virus, SAR-CoV-2, belongs to this virus group, but this is not the same as showing that ivermectin is effective against SAR-CoV-2.

This case highlights ethical issues in how research is reported and used by policymakers. The April study generated much interest in Latin America where ivermectin is used widely for its approved indications. This interest led to many people taking ivermectin for COVID-19, resulting in shortages for its approved uses. The inappropriate use of a limited resource can have far-reaching consequences for others. The *potential* benefit of a drug for a new disease must be balanced against the *actual* benefits that have been demonstrated already.

The resulting shortages led to people using veterinary ivermectin products. This became so widespread that the FDA issued a warning about the different types of products.[19] Then on April 6, 2020, another study was reported as a preprint publication.[20] When researchers submit a manuscript to an academic journal, it undergoes peer review whereby independent researchers evaluate the study to ensure it was conducted rigorously and ethically and reported accurately. Changes may be suggested or required before publication, or the article may be rejected because of weaknesses or a lack of match with the journal's aims. The peer-review process can take months, which is a problem when research is being conducted on urgent topics. For that reason, some journals now allow authors to make their reports available as "preprints" while the peer review process proceeds. This makes the results available to clinicians, policymakers, and others more quickly, but it has to be remembered that such preprints are not peer reviewed. Therefore, they must be carefully evaluated by readers. Various tools are available for this process, technically called critical appraisal.[21]

The ivermectin preprint provided data from a database owned by a U.S. company called Surgisphere.[22] The owner, Dr. Sapan Desai, co-authored this preprint and other publications that will be discussed later. Surgisphere reportedly collected data on COVID-19 patients from hospitals around the world. This preprint reported that patients receiving ivermectin had improved survival rates. The death rate was 18.6% for COVID-19 patients not receiving ivermectin but was 7.7% for those receiving ivermectin. The authors posted a new version of their study a few weeks later in which they compared similar patients with one another (rather than reporting overall averages). This revision found more dramatic differences.[23] Those taking ivermectin had a death rate of 1.4% compared to 8.5% for similar patients not receiving ivermectin.

Ivermectin usage in Latin America increased even further, leading to ethical dilemmas exemplified by Victor Zamora, Peru's Health Minister. As they developed guidelines for clinicians in Peru, Zamora stated that they did not have time "to wait for scientific evidence," while Dr. Eduardo Gotuzzo, a tropical medicine expert, asked, "What do you do?" for seriously ill patients; "Give them water?" implying that a placebo-controlled study would be unethical.[24] Without research results, Peru added ivermectin to its COVID-19 clinical guidelines in May 2020, followed by Bolivia, and later Brazil and Chile.[25] Doctors reported being pressured to prescribe ivermectin, while researchers reported difficulties conducting RCTs because patients did not want to be randomly assigned to a placebo group. Gradually, however, problems with ivermectin started to materialize, resulting in Patricia Garcia, a Peruvian global health researcher, stating, "I think people have lost faith in science . . . and it has been very, very bad for us in Latin America."[26]

Treatment decisions for any new illness are difficult because of uncertainty. The ivermectin case is more tragic because a closer examination of the two studies discussed above revealed some serious problems. Carlos Chaccour is a Venezuelan physician and researcher who worked in the Amazon and with ivermectin for 12 years. He identified serious discrepancies with the Surgisphere data, concluding that their report "was so weird."[27] He noted that 52 patients were reported as receiving ivermectin before it was recommended for COVID-19. Three patients on ventilators were included from African hospitals, but Chaccour noted that only two COVID-19 patients were known in Africa at this time, neither on ventilators. A third patient was later identified, but similarly was not on a ventilator. Chaccour also worked in Africa for many years and questioned whether many African hospitals had the electronic patient record systems that Surgisphere stated they were using. Other serious discrepancies with the Surgisphere data have since been identified and will be discussed later.

Subsequently, a systematic review of ivermectin research reported that after 50 years of widespread laboratory testing, positive lab results using ivermectin against various viruses have not been reproduced in animals or humans.[28] The review concluded that ivermectin is very poorly absorbed into humans and animals, making very high doses necessary, which risks adverse effects. Ivermectin appears to have little or no value in treating COVID-19, but only on October 12, 2020 was it removed from Peru's clinical guidelines.[29] In the intervening months, many people using the drug potentially suffered various adverse effects. The rush to produce research should not justify either premature or questionable publications, and results should always be critiqued before they are used to guide patient-related decisions.

Case 2: Hydroxychloroquine

The second case involves two related drugs, hydroxychloroquine and chloroquine. These are both FDA-approved to prevent and treat malaria. Additionally, hydroxychloroquine is approved to treat some autoimmune disorders and has fewer adverse effects, heightening interest in it compared to chloroquine.[30] Hydroxychloroquine received much media exposure when a study in France reported benefits in March 2020.[31] However, this study's details need to be examined. Only 36 COVID-19 patients were enrolled in this open-label study, meaning that everyone involved knew who received hydroxychloroquine and who did not. Such studies are known to introduce a high risk of bias compared to RCTs where everyone is blinded. In addition, some of the patients receiving hydroxychloroquine also received azithromycin, another drug proposed as a COVID-19 treatment. Providing this drug to some but not all patients further complicates the analysis, making any conclusions about effectiveness very difficult. The principal investigator, Didier Raoult, rejected criticisms of his study, claiming that these represented the "dictatorship of the methodologists."[32] Media interest was sparked, and the Presidents of France and the U.S. got involved.[33] Half a million people in France signed a petition calling for greater access to hydroxychloroquine, supported by a former Minister of Health and one of France's leading infectious disease experts, Professor Christian Perrone. Perrone revealed that he refused to carry out RCTs believing it was unethical to include a placebo group for COVID-19 patients.[34]

Further evidence supporting hydroxychloroquine came from a study in China that became available as a preprint in April 2020.[35] News media quickly reported that COVID-19 patients recovered more quickly when given hydroxychloroquine.[36] One infectious disease expert stated that "it's going to send a ripple of excitement out through the treating community."[37] In accordance with best practices, a protocol, or detailed description of the study methods, was available before the study started. Protocols are increasingly recommended or required to discourage researchers from changing their studies in ways that increase the risk of bias. If changes are required during the study, these should be justified in published reports. Protocols also aim to encourage researchers to publish results, whether positive or negative.

When comparing the preprint with the original protocol, several major changes can be seen.[38] The protocol stated that the study would involve 3 groups of 100 people each receiving either 100 mg hydroxychloroquine twice daily, 200 mg hydroxychloroquine twice daily, or a starch pill (placebo). The published report had the higher dose group, but only one other group and it received standard care (not a placebo). Only 31 participants were in each group, raising questions about whether enough participants enrolled to satisfy statistical requirements. In addition, the protocol planned to recruit people between 30 and 65 years of age, but the report stated only that participants were over 18 years of age. Other significant changes were made and not discussed in the preprint.

These details raise concerns about why the changes were made, how they weakened the rigor of the methods, and the potential bias they introduced. Such issues would normally be addressed during peer review and would highlight how news media and practitioners should not rely on preprints until after they have been evaluated. To date, this study has not been published in a peer-reviewed journal.

Even when studies are published in prestigious peer-reviewed journals, ethical problems can arise. On May 1, 2020, *The New England Journal of Medicine* published a study concluding that patients with heart disease had worse outcomes with COVID-19.[39] Other reports had found similar results, but this study was based on data from almost nine thousand patients in the Surgisphere database discussed earlier. On May 22, the same research group published a study in *Lancet* based on data from almost 100,000 patients in 1,200 hospitals around the world. This study reported that the death rates and incidence of heart problems increased in COVID-19 patients taking hydroxychloroquine.[40] The next day, WHO halted the use of hydroxychloroquine in its large international study called the Solidarity Trial. Other hydroxychloroquine trials were stopped also. One researcher commented that the *Lancet* article's "findings, to many, seemed definitive."[41]

However, closer examination of the two Surgisphere publications showed that they contained data from more Australian COVID-19 patients than existed at that time. This led to *Lancet* publishing a correction.[42] More questions arose about Surgisphere and its founder, Desai, also a co-author on the two big studies. Prior to 2019, Surgisphere was a medical textbook publisher, raising questions about how it could so rapidly become a data analytics and artificial intelligence company.[43] Australian hospitals were contacted about how they contributed patient data, but none had any knowledge of Surgisphere. Investigative journalists noted that data on race was reported for countries where such data is not collected. These and other concerns led all of Desai's co-authors, but not Desai himself, to retract both articles on June 4. The co-authors admitted they had not viewed or analyzed the data themselves. This violates standard principles of publication ethics, exemplified by an article published almost 10 years earlier: "It is incumbent upon the publisher, editors, authors, and readers to ensure that the highest standards of scientific scholarship are upheld."[44]

Researchers must ensure that when putting their names on publications, they know where the data has come from, how the analysis was conducted, and how the findings were developed from that data. An ethical responsibility exists to check everything carefully so that authors know that the claims being made are supported by the data. Editors and peer-reviewers, likewise, have an ethical responsibility to check that the results provided in submitted articles can be verified. Readers and consumers of evidence similarly have an ethical responsibility to critically appraise studies that are used to inform clinical decisions and policies. Just because an article is published in a well-known, peer-reviewed journal should not be enough to accept its conclusions without careful appraisal. Part of the irony of this situation is that Desai was the lead author of the publication quoted at the end of the last paragraph.

The pandemic has put pressure on researchers and publishers to make their research available quickly. While this is important, the urgency to publish must be balanced against the importance of accuracy. If mistakes, or even fraud, get published in the rush to publication, this can harm those who rely on those inaccurate findings and undermine public trust in research and medical science.

These examples highlight one way that research ethics involves much more than ethics approval. The studies conducted in France and China had all the required ethical approvals, and the Surgisphere studies were deemed exempt from ethical review because they involved anonymized, aggregate data. The researchers conformed to ethics regulations, but many other ethical issues remain since these drugs have been used by "hundreds of thousands of patients, but with scant evidence about the risks and benefits."[45]

After the Surgisphere articles were retracted, research involving hydroxychloroquine started up again and publications followed. Enthusiasm for an intervention should not be based on a single trial but should await the clearer picture that develops from a body of research. Clarity has developed with hydroxychloroquine. Systematic reviews summarize the results of several studies, with one review of 24 small hydroxychloroquine studies concluding that the evidence about its effectiveness was weak and conflicting.[46] In June 2020, the RECOVERY trial in the UK, which involved thousands of participants, reported that their data "convincingly rule out any meaningful mortality benefit" from hydroxychloroquine.[47]

Another question with hydroxychloroquine is whether taking it prophylactically prevents infection. Two studies came out in June 2020 reporting no benefit here.[48] Then a large observational study in New York found no benefit from hydroxychloroquine, and the National Institutes of Health (NIH) stopped its large RCT because it found no benefit.[49] As a result of these and other research results, the FDA revoked its emergency use authorization, granted due to the initial public interest and the results of small studies.[50] The WHO also stopped using hydroxychloroquine in its Solidarity Trial. While these studies have found no evidence of harm in patients taking hydroxychloroquine, indirect harm results from hydroxychloroquine being diverted away from its approved uses, resulting in shortages for those who could benefit from those approved uses.

In spite of these results, "the pressure to *do something* is enormous and understandable" for those caring for COVID-19 patients.[51] Giving in to public pressure is not the ethical way forward. Healthcare professionals need to remain focused on the available evidence and work against rumors and misinformation. The ethical way to respond to uncertainty and fear is to "inform patients about the evidence behind experimental therapies, work to enroll patients in randomized clinical trials, and consider the needs of patients without COVID-19 who may be effected by drug shortages."[52]

Case 3: Remdesivir

The third case highlights how research can contribute during a pandemic. Remdesivir became the first FDA-approved treatment for COVID-19 on October 22, 2020.[53] Prior to COVID-19, it showed promise against two other coronavirus diseases, SARS and MERS, and had shown encouraging results in animal and laboratory studies.[54] This previous research was quickly adapted to COVID-19.

A large RCT called the ACTT-1 Trial enrolled patients with COVID-19 who had respiratory problems and were more seriously ill.[55] After enrolling over 1,000 patients, their safety monitoring committee stopped the trial because it was clear that patients receiving Remdesivir were benefiting.[56] Those taking a placebo took an average of 15 days to recover, while those taking Remdesivir took 11 days. The mortality rate showed a positive trend, going from 11.9% to 7.1% with Remdesivir, but this was not statistically significant. They also found that the most seriously ill patients, those on ventilators, did not benefit from the drug. The trial was stopped for ethical reasons: so that all patients would have the opportunity to receive Remdesivir.

A methodologically rigorous trial like ACTT-1 shows differences between groups of patients and can thus provide clear evidence that can guide practice and highlight important differences between groups of patients. Other researchers reported that "Conducting such a clinical trial only a few months after SARS-CoV-2 was discovered is an extraordinary achievement."[57]

Doing a trial of this type raises all the usual ethical issues with clinical research in the midst of a pandemic. This trial had additional ethical issues because very little drug was available when the research started. Very few patients could be invited to participate in the trial, which required ways to ethically allocate those invitations justly and fairly. However, even as those policies were put in place, further research pointed to new evidence that allowed more patients to receive the drug. The initial protocol for Remdesivir provided the drug for 10 days. When results showed that a 5-day course was as effective as 10 days, twice as many people could be enrolled.[58]

Flexibility within trials is part of a more general approach to RCTs called "adaptive designs," exemplified by the WHO Solidarity Trial. This approach developed in response to criticisms that RCTs can be overly rigid and inflexible, insisting on continuing on to the planned endpoints rather than adapting as conditions change. In an adaptive trial design, plans to change and adapt are built into the trial from the beginning.[59] This adds additional complexity to the trial design, and requires additional statistical expertise to interpret results. However, it allows rigor to be maintained, even as researchers respond to the urgency and seriousness of the pandemic.

The Solidarity Trial has enrolled more than 11,000 participants at 405 hospitals in 30 countries.[60] About 100 countries are interested in becoming involved. In addition, the WHO is assisting 60 low-income countries with obtaining IRB approval, providing training for researchers and clinicians, and getting access to the experimental drugs. Not only is this right and just, but it allows people from different backgrounds and settings to become participants, not just those from wealthy countries. As a result, Solidarity should provide a truly global picture of the efficacy of these drugs.

To complicate the overall picture for Remdesivir, Solidarity's interim analysis concluded that Remdesivir provided no benefit to COVID-19 patients. As a result of this and other trials, WHO has since recommended against its use.[61] This contrasts with the ACCT-1 results, and the FDA recommendation. Unfortunately, the uncertainty continues, but this is part of the challenge with a novel illness. In addition, research into a new intervention sometimes produces inconsistent evidence at first, and over time a clearer picture emerges about its effectiveness and whether particular patients benefit more or less.

Case 4: COVID-19 Vaccines

The fourth case involves vaccines being developed for COVID-19. Many are placing their hopes for overcoming this pandemic on a vaccine. However, it must be remembered that "vaccine development is a lengthy, expensive process. Attrition is high, and it typically takes multiple candidates and many years to produce a licensed vaccine."[62] A huge amount of research is being carried out in this area. As of November 21, 2020, 260 vaccine candidates exist, with 56 in clinical testing of which 11 are in Phase III trials, the last before being licensed.[63] This is remarkable progress within less than a year of COVID-19 being declared a pandemic. It now appears that a vaccine will be available before the end of 2020.

Previously, the fastest a vaccine was developed was five years for Ebola. To get so far so quickly, phases that are normally sequential are being overlapped.[64] However, this carries risks, some of which are financial. The Gates Foundation is spending billions on constructing seven factories, knowing that only one or two of them may ever be used for COVID-19 vaccines because they may not be suitable for the vaccines eventually developed.[65]

Other risks are more specifically linked to research ethics, two of which will be addressed here.[66] First, given how rapidly vaccine trials are being developed, the time to watch for adverse reactions will be shortened. Typically, more basic research is conducted to understand a virus and the illness it causes, but less time has passed to do this with SARS-CoV-2 and COVID-19. Initiating later trial phases sooner means that less time has been taken to identify adverse effects, some of which may take months or years to develop. Innovative processes are being used, such as a new class of vaccines called messenger RNA vaccines. While this has novel benefits, such as allowing more rapid development, unknown risks may be involved.

All research carries some risk of harm, especially clinical trials involving experimental interventions. This is addressed ethically through a complex process of balancing harms and benefits. The harms caused by COVID-19 are clear, both for individuals and societies. Taking higher risks than normal can be justified. This requires transparency and honesty in communicating both with potential trial participants and the public. Known risks with any vaccine candidate should be communicated as part of the informed consent process for both trials and administration of the vaccine. COVID-19 vaccine trials also require that uncertainty about risks and benefits, especially any atypical steps during the research process, should be communicated clearly. This is ethically crucial to respect those volunteering to take experimental vaccines, but it is also vital for public trust in any vaccine that becomes available. Researchers and vaccine developers may be tempted to overlook adverse effects, which is why independent bodies of experts are involved in reviewing data at various stages. Hence, two prominent COVID-19 vaccine trials were halted because of unexplained adverse events.[67] This is tragic for those participants, and discouraging overall, yet must be done to ensure the research is ethically robust.

A second ethical issue with COVID-19 vaccine research is the use of challenge trials. These involve healthy volunteers who receive the experimental vaccines and then are exposed deliberately to the virus or a modified form of it. Some argue that it is unethical to deliberately expose research subjects to this form of increased risk.[68] The principle of risk parity has been proposed to justify challenge trials. Advocates point out that people like healthcare workers caring for COVID-19 patients take on increased risks of harm in order to benefit others.[69] In a similar way, fully informed volunteers should be permitted to accept additional risks in research.[70] Challenge trials have occurred with other vaccines, but these involved well-understood diseases for which treatments were available if the candidate vaccine does not work and people become ill. In contrast, COVID-19 is new and poorly understood, and effective treatments are only now becoming available. Volunteers would most likely be healthy and young, and thus not in the high-risk categories for COVID-19. However, people of all ages have died from COVID-19, so they would be putting themselves at some increased risk.

The key ethical issue again comes down to informing potential participants of the risks, known and unknown. Honesty and transparency must be promoted. At the same time, participation in challenge trials must be truly voluntary. Participants must not be required to accept these risks through either open or subtle coercion. This may be particularly challenging if volunteers are sought from healthcare workers who may feel pressured into such trials as part of some duty. Similarly, underprivileged participants should not become participants because they believe this is the only avenue by which they can obtain a vaccine. Researchers will need to work diligently to avoid such pressures. A caveat here is that challenge trials may not be needed if the pandemic continues to spread widely and people are regularly exposed to the virus naturally.

Resource Allocation

A safe and effective COVID-19 vaccine will bring many benefits, but it will also raise additional ethical challenges. Any vaccine will be available in limited quantities at first, which raises questions about how it will be distributed justly and fairly. Both the U.S. National Academies and WHO have proposed allocation schemes whereby vaccines will be allocated fairly.[71] The two prioritization schemes are very similar, putting healthcare workers caring for COVID-19 patients at the top of the list, with high-risk individuals, such as older people with comorbidities, next.

COVID-19 adds an extra level of allocation decisions because of the global nature of the pandemic. Wealthy countries have the resources to purchase large quantities of vaccines immediately, which has already happened. This could leave little or none available for low-income countries until much later. Their populations could continue to suffer disproportionately while the wealthy benefit from the vaccine. Even within countries, unfair allocation could permit wealthier people to purchase vaccines while those living in slums, refugee camps, or other low-income settings are left unprotected.

The WHO is co-leading a consortium called COVID-19 Vaccines Global Access (or COVAX) to address issues of global justice in COVID-19 vaccines and treatments.[72] In this arrangement, wealthier countries contribute to a global fund to purchase vaccines. When the vaccine becomes available, low-income countries will be able to obtain the vaccines along with wealthier countries. As part of joining COVAX, all countries agree to follow the same distribution scheme. As of November 2020, 186 countries have committed to COVAX, 92 low-income countries and 94 higher-income countries.[73] The U.S. was one of the few countries in the world which was not involved, although this changed under President Biden. When vaccines become available, all countries will receive enough vaccine for 3% of their populations, which should allow all healthcare workers to be vaccinated.[74] As more vaccine becomes available, countries will receive enough for 20% of their populations to cover high-risk people. After that, vaccines will be distributed according to the needs in each region.

Underlying these allocation schemes is the growing focus on the ethical principle of solidarity. This has been defined as an "'enacted commitment to carry 'costs' (financial, social, emotional, or otherwise) to assist others with whom a person or persons recognize similarity in a relevant respect.'"[75] This goes beyond empathy to action based on a commitment to others. For example, the cost of participating in a challenge trial (in terms of increased risk) can be seen as an expression of solidarity with those at risk from the disease. Solidarity also aims to base the commitment to action on similarities. Rather than focusing on differences between groups, solidarity points to how we are all in this together and how we need to unite to address the challenges we face.

Applying Biblical Wisdom

Solidarity has been critiqued because "our sense of solidarity is strongest when those with whom solidarity is expressed are thought of as 'one of us.'"[76] Such a view of solidarity would lead to a neglect of those with whom we have little sense of solidarity. This can even lead to unfair distribution if "our group" is given inappropriate preference.

Biblical wisdom provides important input here. Respect for all humans is firmly based in how all are made in the image and likeness of God (Gen 1:26–27; cf. James 3:9). This leads to a commitment to overcome the barriers that keep us separated. "There is neither Jew nor Greek, slave nor free, male nor female, for you are all one in Christ Jesus" (Gal 3:28, NIV). The equal value of all people should lead to a commitment to help others. Galatians 6:2 is just one passage identifying the importance of this in the Bible: "Carry each other's burdens, and in this way you will fulfill the law of Christ."

The concern within global justice to distribute resources equitably overlaps well with the biblical concern for those who are vulnerable. "Defend the cause of the weak and fatherless; maintain the rights of the poor and oppressed. Rescue the weak and needy; deliver them from the hand of the wicked" (Psalm 82:3–4). Generosity is repeatedly praised in the Bible. "If anyone has material possessions and sees his brother in need but closes his heart against him, how can the love of God be in him? Dear children, let us not love with words or tongue but with action and in truth" (1 John 3:17–18).

Knowing the right thing to do includes living life in an authentic way. Scripture provides direct guidance here, but we can also learn from observing nature. The Bible encourages us to learn from the natural world which reveals aspects of God's character qualities (Romans 1:20). When

Daniel and his friends were told by God to follow a specific diet while imprisoned in Babylon, they urged the Babylonians to observe their health as time passed (Daniel 1:12–13). The Babylonians were skeptical at first, but were convinced by the results of this trial. Clearly not a controlled trial, the story points to the value in observing the natural course of events, carefully recording what is seen, and basing conclusions on these results.

The four cases reported here highlight the importance of critically appraising literature. In the book of Acts, the people of the Berea were praised for carefully evaluating Paul's sermons. While they were enthusiastic about what he said, they carefully checked his teaching against the Scriptures (Acts 17:11). Likewise, we should check what we read, whether from theological, medical, or media sources. God gives us evidence to support our beliefs, but we must examine that evidence to evaluate its accuracy and reliability, as Luke carefully investigated his sources as he wrote his gospel (Luke 1:1-4). This ties into the biblical commitment to being truthful, honest, and reliable.

Conclusion

As the COVID-19 pandemic continues, research is a key element of the response. Treatments and vaccines will be important in overcoming the challenges currently faced. That research must be conducted ethically. Those who use the results of that research also have ethical responsibilities. In all stages of research, transparency is crucial. Patients should be informed when interventions have uncertain benefits and harms. If they are experimental, this should be expressed clearly by clinicians and also in the media. Such interventions need further research which should be conducted with rigorous methods. Controlled studies are needed to answer efficacy and effectiveness questions, but at the same time other studies are needed to address other types of questions.

Flexibility is also important, but it has to be introduced appropriately. Ethics approval procedures can take long periods of time, so changes may be needed during a pandemic. For example, some ethics committees have been meeting daily rather than monthly to facilitate rigorous review in timely ways. The speed at which protocols are approved must be balanced against the risk of harm to participants and patients if overly risky research is allowed to proceed.

During the research process, data should be collected and disseminated accurately, with conclusions based on the results and not hyped. Readers and users of evidence also need to appraise reports carefully. Particular attention is needed to preprints and press releases. Research results need to be made available in timely ways, but this must be balanced against the importance of ensuring the accuracy and rigor of what is published.

As treatments and vaccines become available, justice and fairness are crucial in allocation decisions. The global implications of such decisions must be taken into account. As the world struggles to deal with this pandemic, uncertainty is likely to continue in many areas. This means that humility is very important. We need to base decisions on the best-available evidence, acknowledging the limitations of that evidence and where we have no evidence to guide us. If we don't know something, we should admit that we don't know. Because of the lack of evidence, mistakes will be made and guidelines will change. This is unfortunately the case in many areas around COVID-19. It requires communication that is honest and transparent as a way to respect individuals and communities as we all grapple with this challenging situation.

Notes

1. David E. Gordon et al., "A SARS-CoV-2 Protein Interaction Map Reveals Targets for Drug Repurposing," *Nature* 583 (2020): 459, https://doi.org/10.1038/s41586-020-2286-9.

2. Lawrence Corey, John R. Mascola, Anthony S. Fauci, and Francis S. Collins, "A Strategic Approach to COVID-19 Vaccine R&D," *Science* 368, no. 6494 (2020): 948. https://doi.org/10.1126/science.abc5312.

3. WHO, *A Coordinated Global Research Roadmap: 2019 Novel Coronavirus* (Geneva: WHO, March 2020), 4, https://www.who.int/blueprint/priority-diseases/key-action/Coronavirus_Roadmap_V9.pdf.

4. WHO, *A Coordinated Global Research Roadmap*.

5. Alfred H. J. Kim et al., "A Rush to Judgment? Rapid Reporting and Dissemination of Results and Its Consequences Regarding the Use of Hydroxychloroquine for COVID-19," *Annals of Internal Medicine* 172, no. 12 (2020): 820, https://doi.org/10.7326/M20-1223.

6. National Academies of Sciences, Engineering, and Medicine, *Evidence-Based Practice for Public Health Emergency Preparedness and Response* (Washington, DC: The National Academies Press, 2020), https://doi.org/10.17226/25650.

7. Jennifer Couzin-Frankel, "'We've Got to Be Able to Move More Quickly.' The Pandemic Reality of COVID-19 Clinical Trials," *Science*, June 16, 2020, https://doi.org/10.1126/science.abd3588.

8. Jonathan Kimmelman and Alex John London, "Predicting Harms and Benefits in Translational Trials: Ethics, Evidence, and Uncertainty," *PLOS Medicine* 8, no. 3 (2011): 1, https://doi.org/10.1371/journal.pmed.1001010.

9. Couzin-Frankel, "'We've Got to Be Able to Move More Quickly.'"

10. Alex John London and Jonathan Kimmelman, "Against Pandemic Exceptionalism," *Science* 368, no. 6490 (2020): 476–77, https://doi.org/10.1126/science.abc1731.

11. Daniel B. Chastain et al., "Racial Disproportionality in Covid Clinical Trials," *The New England Journal of Medicine* 383, no. 9 (2020), e59, https://doi.org/10.1056/NEJMp2021971.

12. Dónal O'Mathúna and Chesmal Siriwardhana, "Research Ethics and Evidence for Humanitarian Health," *The Lancet* 390, no. 10,109 (2017): 2228–29, https://doi.org/10.1016/S0140-6736(17)31276-X.

13. Dónal O'Mathúna, "The Dual Imperative in Disaster Research Ethics,"

in *SAGE Handbook of Qualitative Research Ethics*, ed. Ron Iphofen and Martin Tolich (London: SAGE, 2018), 441–54.

14. Dónal O'Mathúna. "How Should Clinicians Engage with Online Health Information?" *AMA Journal of Ethics* 20, no. 11 (2018): E1059-E1066, https://doi.org/10.1001/amajethics.2018.1059.

15. Carlos Chaccour, Felix Hammann, Santiago Ramón-Garcín, and N. Regina Rabinovich, "Ivermectin and COVID-19: Keeping Rigor in Times of Urgency," *The American Journal of Tropical Medicine and Hygiene* 102, no. 6 (2020): 1156–57, https://doi.org/10.4269/ajtmh.20-0271.

16. Leon Caly et al., "The FDA-Approved Drug Ivermectin Inhibits the Replication of SARS-CoV-2 *in vitro*," *Antiviral Research* 178, no. 104,787 (2020): https://doi.org/10.1016/j.antiviral.2020.104787.

17. Aila Slisco. "Anti-Parasite Drug Used Since 1980s May Help Stop Coronavirus, New Study Says," *Newsweek*, April 3, 2020, https://www.newsweek.com/anti-parasite-drug-used-since-1980s-may-help-stop-coronavirus-new-study-says-1496083.

18. Chaccour, Hammann, Ramón-Garcín, and Rabinovich, "Ivermectin and COVID-19."

19. Steven Solomon, "FDA Letter to Stakeholders: Do Not Use Ivermectin Intended for Animals as Treatment for COVID-19 in Humans," U.S. FDA, April 10, 2020, https://www.fda.gov/animal-veterinary/product-safety-information/fda-letter-stakeholders-do-not-use-ivermectin-intended-animals-treatment-covid-19-humans.

20. Amit N.Patel, Sapan S. Desai, David W. Grainger, and Mandeep R. Mehra, Ivermectin in COVID-19 Related Critical Illness," ISGlobal.org, 2020, https://www.isglobal.org/documents/10179/6022921/Patel+et+al.+2020+version+1.pdf/fab19388-dc3e-4593-a075-db96f4536e9d (accessed December 3, 2020; Retracted).

21. Critical Appraisal Skills Program, "CASP Checklists," CASP-UK.net, 2019, https://casp-uk.net/casp-tools-checklists/ (accessed December 3, 2020).

22. Catherine Offord, "Surgisphere Sows Confusion about Another Unproven COVID-19 Drug," *The Scientist,* June 16, 2020, https://www.the-scientist.com/news-opinion/surgisphere-sows-confusion-about-another-unproven-covid19-drug-67635.

23. Amit N.Patel, Sapan S. Desai, David W. Grainger, and Mandeep R. Mehra, "Usefulness of Ivermectin in COVID-19 Illness," ISGlobal.org, April 20, 2020, https://www.isglobal.org/documents/10179/6022921/Patel+et+al.+2020+version+2.pdf/adf390e0-7099-4c70-91d0-e0f7a0b69e14

(Retracted).

24. Offord, "Surgisphere Sows Confusion about Another Unproven COVID-19 Drug."

25. Melissa Davey, "Unreliable Data: How Doubt Snowballed over Covid-19 Drug Research That Swept the World," *The Guardian*, June 4, 2020, https://www.theguardian.com/world/2020/jun/04/unreliable-data-doubt-snowballed-covid-19-drug-research-surgisphere-coronavirus-hydroxychloroquine.

26. Offord, "Surgisphere Sows Confusion about Another Unproven COVID-19 Drug."

27. Davey, "Unreliable Data;" Offord, "Surgisphere Sows Confusion about Another Unproven COVID-19 Drug."

28. Fatemeh Heidary and Reza Gharebaghi, "Ivermectin: A Systematic Review from Antiviral Effects to COVID-19 Complementary Regimen," *The Journal of Antibiotics* 73, no. 9 (2020): 593–602, https://doi.org/10.1038/s41429-020-0336-z.

29. Catherine Offord, "Surgisphere Sows Confusion about Another Unproven COVID-19 Drug: Update," *The Scientist*, October 13, 2020, https://www.the-scientist.com/news-opinion/surgisphere-sows-confusion-about-another-unproven-covid19-drug-67635.

30. Philippe Gautret et al., "Hydroxychloroquine and Azithromycin as a Treatment of COVID-19: Results of an Open-Label Non-Randomized Clinical Trial," *International Journal of Antimicrobial Agents* 56, no. 1 (2020): https://doi.org/10.1016/j.ijantimicag.2020.105949.

31. Gautret et al., "Hydroxychloroquine and Azithromycin as a Treatment of COVID-19."

32. Yves Sciama, "Is France's President Fueling the Hype over an Unproven Coronavirus Treatment?" *Science*, April 9, 2020, https://www.sciencemag.org/news/2020/04/france-s-president-fueling-hype-over-unproven-coronavirus-treatment.

33. Sciama, "Is France's President Fueling the Hype over an Unproven Coronavirus Treatment?"

34. Sciama, "Is France's President Fueling the Hype over an Unproven Coronavirus Treatment?"

35. Zhaowei Chen et al., "Efficacy of Hydroxychloroquine in Patients with COVID-19: Results of a Randomized Clinical Trial," *MedRxIV* (April 10, 2020): https://doi.org/10.1101/2020.03.22.20040758.

36. Denise Grady, "Malaria Drug Helps Virus Patients Improve, in Small Study," *New York Times*, April 1, 2020, https://www.nytimes.com/2020/04/01/health/hydroxychloroquine-coronavirus-malaria.html.

37. Grady, "Malaria Drug Helps Virus Patients Improve, in Small Study."

38. Robin E. Ferner and Jeffrey K. Aronson, "Hydroxychloroquine for COVID-19: What Do the Clinical Trials Tell Us?" Centre for Evidence-Based Medicine, April 14, 2020, https://www.cebm.net/covid-19/hydroxychloroquine-for-covid-19-what-do-the-clinical-trials-tell-us/.

39. Mandeep R. Mehra et al., "Cardiovascular Disease, Drug Therapy, and Mortality in Covid-19," *The New England Journal of Medicine* 382, no. 25 (2020): e102, https://doi.org/10.1056/NEJMoa2007621 (Retracted).

40. Mandeep R. Mehra, Sapan S. Desai, Frank Ruschitzka, and Amit N Patel, "Hydroxychloroquine or Chloroquine with or without a Macrolide for Treatment of COVID-19: A Multinational Registry Analysis," *The Lancet* (May 22, 2020): https://doi.org/10.1016/S0140-6736(20)31180-6 (Retracted).

41. Davey, "Unreliable Data."

42. "Department of Error," *The Lancet* (May 30, 2020): https://doi.org/10.1016/S0140-6736(20)31249-6.

43. Melissa Davey and Stephanie Kirchgaessner, "Surgisphere: Mass Audit of Papers Linked to Firm behind Hydroxychloroquine *Lancet* Study Scandal," *The Guardian*, June 10, 2020, https://www.theguardian.com/world/2020/jun/10/surgisphere-sapan-desai-lancet-study-hydroxychloroquine-mass-audit-scientific-papers.

44. Sapan S. Desai and Cynthia K. Shortell, "Conflicts of Interest for Medical Publishers and Editors: Protecting the Integrity of Scientific Scholarship," *Journal of Vascular Surgery* 54, no. 3 supplement (2011): 59S-63S, https://doi.org/10.1016/j.jvs.2011.05.111.

45. Eric J. Rubin et al., "The Urgency of Care during the Covid-19 Pandemic—Learning as We Go," *The New England Journal of Medicine* 382, no. 25 (2020): 2461–2, https://doi.org/10.1056/NEJMe2015903.

46. Adrian V. Hernandez et al., "Hydroxychloroquine or Chloroquine for Treatment or Prophylaxis of COVID-19: A Living Systematic Review," *Annals of Internal Medicine* 173, no. 4 (2020): 287–96, https://doi.org/10.7326/M20-2496.

47. Peter Horby and Martin Landray, "No Clinical Benefit from Use of Hydroxychloroquine in Hospitalised Patients with COVID-19," *RECOVERY*, June 5, 2020, https://www.recoverytrial.net/news/statement-from-the-chief-investigators-of-the-randomised-evaluation-of-covid-19-therapy-recovery-trial-on-hydroxychloroquine-5-june-2020-no-clinical-benefit-from-use-of-hydroxychloroquine-in-hospitalised-patients-with-covid-19.

48. Katie Thomas, "Federal Agency Halts Studies of Hydroxychloroquine,

Drug Trump Promoted," *The New York Times*, June 20, 2020, https://www.nytimes.com/2020/06/20/health/hydroxychloroquine-coronavirus-trial.html.

49. National Department of Health & Human Services, "NIH Halts Clinical Trial of Hydroxychloroquine," NIH, June 20, 2020. https://www.nih.gov/news-events/news-releases/nih-halts-clinical-trial-hydroxychloroquine.

50. Joshua Geleris et al., "Observational Study of Hydroxychloroquine in Hospitalized Patients with Covid-19," *The New England Journal of Medicine* 382, no. 25 (2020): 2411–18, https://doi.org/10.1056/NEJMoa2012410.

51. Colette DeJong and Robert M. Wachter, "The Risks of Prescribing Hydroxychloroquine for Treatment of COVID-19—First, Do No Harm," *JAMA Internal Medicine* 180, no. 8 (2020): 1118, https://doi.org/10.1001/jamainternmed.2020.1853 (emphasis original).

52. DeJong and Wachter, "The Risks of Prescribing Hydroxychloroquine for Treatment of COVID-19," 1118.

53. "FDA Approves First Treatment for COVID-19," U.S. FDA, October 22, 2020, https://www.fda.gov/news-events/press-announcements/fda-approves-first-treatment-covid-19.

54. J. H. Beigel et al., "Remdesivir for the Treatment of Covid-19—Final Report," *The New England Journal of Medicine* 383, no. 19 (2020): 1813–26, https://doi.org/10.1056/NEJMoa2007764.

55. Beigel et al., "Remdesivir for the Treatment of Covid-19."

56. Beigel et al., "Remdesivir for the Treatment of Covid-19."

57. Raphael Dolin and Martin S. Hirsch, "Remdesivir—An Important First Step," *The New England Journal of Medicine* 383, no. 19 (2020): 1886, https://doi.org/10.1056/NEJMe2018715.

58. Jason D. Goldman et al., "Remdesivir for 5 or 10 Days in Patients with Severe Covid-19," *The New England Journal of Medicine* 383, no. 19 (2020): 1827–37, https://doi.org/10.1056/NEJMoa2015301.

59. Philip Pallmann et al., "Adaptive Designs in Clinical Trials: Why Use Them, and How to Run and Report Them," *BMC Medicine* 16, no. 29 (2018): https://doi.org/10.1186/s12916-018-1017-7.

60. WHO Solidarity Trial Consortium, "Repurposed Antiviral Drugs for COVID-19—Interim WHO SOLIDARITY Trial Results," *MedRxIV* (October 15, 2020): https://doi.org/10.1101/2020.10.15.20209817.

61. Benedict Carey, "W.H.O. Rejects Antiviral Drug Remdesivir as a Covid Treatment," *The New York Times*, November 19, 2020, https://www.nytimes.com/2020/11/19/health/remdesivir-covid-19.html.

62. Nicole Lurie, Melanie Saville, Richard Hatchett, and Jane Halton, "Developing Covid-19 Vaccines at Pandemic Speed," *The New England Journal of Medicine* 382, no. 21 (2020): 1970, https://doi.org/10.1056/NEJMp2005630.

63. Vaccine Centre, "Vaccine Tracker," London School of Hygiene & Tropical Medicine, November 21, 2020, https://vac-lshtm.shinyapps.io/ncov_vaccine_landscape/.

64. Stuart A. Thompson, "How Long Will a Vaccine Really Take?" *The New York Times*, April 30, 2020, https://www.nytimes.com/interactive/2020/04/30/opinion/coronavirus-covid-vaccine.html.

65. Isobel Asher Hamilton, "Bill Gates Is Funding New Factories for Potential Coronavirus Vaccines," World Economic Forum, April 6, 2020, https://www.weforum.org/agenda/2020/04/bill-gates-7-potential-coronavirus-vaccines.

66. Lurie et al., "Developing Covid-19 Vaccines at Pandemic Speed;" Thompson, "How Long Will a Vaccine Really Take?"

67. Carl Zimmer, "3 Covid-19 Trials Have Been Paused for Safety. That's a Good Thing," *The New York Times*, October 14, 2020, https://www.nytimes.com/2020/10/14/health/covid-clinical-trials.html.

68. Jon Cohen, "Speed Coronavirus Vaccine Testing by Deliberately Infecting Volunteers? Not so Fast, Some Scientists Warn," *Science*, March 31, 2020, https://doi.org/10.1126/science.abc0006.

69. Richard Yetter Chappell and Peter Singer, "Pandemic Ethics: The Case for Risky Research," *Research Ethics* 16, no. 3–4 (2020): 1–8, https://doi.org/10.1177/1747016120931920.

70. Stanley A. Plotkin, "Extraordinary Diseases Require Extraordinary Solutions," *Vaccine* 38 (2020): 3987–88, https://doi.org/10.1016/j.vaccine.2020.04.039.

71. National Academies of Sciences, Engineering, and Medicine, *Framework for Equitable Allocation of COVID-19 Vaccine* (Washington, DC: The National Academies Press, 2020), https://doi.org/10.17226/25917; WHO, "Fair Allocation Mechanism for COVID-19 Vaccines through the COVAX Facility," WHO.int, September 9, 2020, https://www.who.int/publications/m/item/fair-allocation-mechanism-for-covid-19-vaccines-through-the-covax-facility.

72. WHO, "COVAX: Working for Global Equitable Access to COVID-19 Vaccines," WHO.int, https://www.who.int/initiatives/act-accelerator/covax (accessed December 4, 2020).

73. Kai Kupferschmidt, WHO Unveils Global Plan to Fairly Distribute COVID-19 Vaccine, But Challenges Await," *Science*, September 21, 2020,

MORAL INJURY IN THE TIME OF COVID-19

JOSEPH WIINIKKA-LYDON

Articles and studies have already begun to assess the psychological impact of the COVID-19 pandemic on healthcare professionals and patients. One term in particular that has not appeared much in healthcare literature or bioethics has become more marked in both journalism and scholarly reflections of the crisis. Originally coined to describe the experiences of soldiers and veterans, *moral injury* points to the way in which people can feel like they are no longer able to strive to be a good person because of what they have done, or failed to do, in wartime. Although I am hesitant to join others in calling the pandemic a war and to associate healthcare professionals with soldiers in combat, the high stakes situations, resource depletion, and challenges such healthcare professionals are facing in the time of COVID-19 do create serious life and death situations that strain one both physically and spiritually in a way that one could rightfully say is injurious to one's character or sense of self. Further, this recent use of moral injury in bioethics will most likely mark a beginning, and not an end. We will see this term used more and more during and after the pandemic to describe experiences whose moral valence other terms and discourses, such as post-traumatic stress disorder (PTSD) and trauma, do not seem to capture fully.

Not surprisingly, recent writings attempting to explore the experience of the pandemic through the lens of moral injury do so, by and large, by taking on the strengths of moral injury discourse as it is found in the psychological literature. In doing so, however, they also reflect some important limitations and uncritical assumptions found in that literature's seminal writings. In particular, there is a general reticence to address broader politics, both in terms of policy making and the politics of wider culture, that condition and shape experiences of moral injury and in which such experiences are inevitably embedded. During normal times, such a broader political analysis may not always be strictly necessary to understand moral injury in a healthcare setting. The current pandemic, however, has been enmeshed from the start with political debates and discourse. Whether one looks at the politicization of mask wearing, policies around statewide closures and curfews, or public opinions on social distancing, the political divides in the United States, its ongoing culture wars, as well as President Trump's administration's highly partisan and polarizing response to the pandemic, have significantly influenced national, statewide, and local approaches to dealing with the pandemic.[1]

In this way, such a pandemic is not simply a matter of medicine. It is inherently political, and so the experience—and injury—of healthcare workers during the pandemic has also been shaped profoundly by politics on many levels. This requires authors of healthcare ethics and bioethics writings who employ moral injury to think more deeply and critically about the ways such injuries may be shaped not just by the pressures one might expect from a pandemic but also by the political context and political responses associated with, or occurring alongside, that pandemic. This is critical, as such reflection will help those engaged in bioethics and healthcare ethics better understand the multifaceted and complex nature of moral injuries, opening up a more nuanced discussion about how we can begin to address the causes of such injuries and their possible repair.

My argument is that there is a critical lacuna emerging in discussions of moral injury and the pandemic. This lacuna arises from the adoption of moral injury research that originates from wartime contexts—the same contexts from which moral injury was first conceptualized. As some researchers have already critically noted, seminal definitions used in psychological research elide the important political contexts that condition such injury.[2] This is important, since the way moral injury is conceptualized influences those therapies developed to heal moral harms. Adopting definitions of moral injury from psychology without addressing such deficits, then, threatens to skew our understanding of the nature of lasting harms that come from crises, such as the current pandemic, and the way we respond to pandemic moral injury.

The goal of the following pages, then, is to intervene early in the adoption of moral injury in bioethics and healthcare ethics so that any understanding of such injury reflects the important political dimension of these moral harms. I engage, first, seminal definitions and understandings of moral injury to illuminate not only their strengths but their deficits when it comes to including politics and culture as factors in moral injury. This will include engaging the discourse of moral distress found in healthcare and nursing ethics. I then draw out the lacunae in both discourses, offering ways to rethink moral injury that may be better able to attend to the multifaceted sources of moral injury.

Moral injury is an important subject for bioethics and broader healthcare ethics, including medical ethics and nursing ethics, to engage. It will not only help descriptively to articulate the experiences of professional healthcare workers. It can also serve as a critical concept to challenge current frames, such as moral distress, that are more common in the healthcare ethics literature, so we may better understand the changes in subjectivity that can occur during the everyday labor of healthcare. As bioethics and healthcare ethics begin to adopt moral injury discourse, then, such adoptions should be done critically and in a way that helps us better understand the complex political dimensions of such injury.

Moral Injury: An Overview

Moral injury is a relatively new concept in healthcare studies and related ethics. Indeed, it is a new concept in general, having been coined by Jonathan Shay, a psychiatrist, in the early 1990s. Shay developed the idea of moral injury while working with U.S. veterans of the wars in Vietnam and Southeast Asia.[3] What Shay argues is that there is a form of harm that veterans described that was not satisfactorily addressed by formal definitions of PTSD. In the *Diagnostic and Statistical Manual*, v 5, published through the American Psychiatric Association, PTSD is categorized as a "stress-related disorder" arising from witnessing, hearing about, or experiencing a traumatic event that results in reliving that event, avoidance, mood changes, hyperarousal, and hypervigilance.[4]

Moral injury's exact relationship to PTSD is still debated. Those who claim that moral injury is something distinct argue that, while PTSD describes a problem with one's cognition and emotional life due to encounters with violence and threat, moral injury gets at an even more amorphous claim, as the undoing of one's sense of moral ability and worldview.[5] While PTSD is seen as an experience of violence that affects one's everyday reaction to events and stimuli, moral injury was coined to express feelings of guilt, shame, anger, and despair arising from one's participation in violence, particularly within a combat environment.

Moral Injury   vs   PTSD

Moral Injury	PTSD
• Participation in violence or allowing something unjust to happen	• "actual or threatened death, serious injury, or sexual violence"
• Violence evaluated to be unjust or to have violated core notions of what is good and right	• Avoidance
	• Flashbacks
• Relatively clear memory of events and a negative evaluation of them	• Prolonged distress, negativity, shame, guilt
• Perceived transformation of identity	• Memory, even language loss and change
• Perceived transformation of character	• Hyper-arousal, aggression, recklessness

Figure 1

There are, however, a variety of definitions for moral injury. Hodgson and Cary, for example, list 12 definitions of wartime moral injury as of 2015, and we could include many more besides.[6] Even so, there are two seminal definitions of moral injury that have developed and that ground subsequent definitions. First, Jonathan Shay's definition has been influential especially in the humanities. Shay argues that moral injury arises when "there has been a betrayal of what's right [to the soldier] by someone who holds legitimate authority in a high-stakes situation."[7] The emphasis here is on a sense of betrayal where the commission or source of moral injury comes from the institution of the military chain of command. According to Shay's original definition, soldiers feel that their trust in leadership has been undermined in a context where one's life and the lives of others are on the line. In other words, they feel betrayed by those in whom they had institutionally placed their trust when lives were on the line.

The second definition originated in a 2009 article by psychologist Brett Litz and his co-authors. This definition has been influential in some humanities work but especially in psychology and the behavioral sciences. The authors argue that moral injury arises from discrete moments or events, "morally injurious events," where a soldier transgresses "deeply held moral beliefs and expectations."[8] This definition emphasizes neither betrayal (except for a sense of self betrayal) nor the institutional context of the military chain of command. Instead, the soldier is both the location of moral injury and also the commissioner, as it is the soldier who violates her own most deeply held values. High-stakes situations are not emphasized, as one can also get moral injury from seeing the aftermath of battle, including seeing dead bodies, or handling remains.[9] It is, then, a much more capacious definition than Shay's.

Shay (1st wave)	Litz et al. (2nd wave)
"Moral injury is present when 1. there has been a betrayal of what's right [in the soldier's eyes] 2. by someone who holds legitimate authority 3. in a high-stakes situation."	Moral injury is caused by: 1. "Potentially morally injurious events, such as perpetrating, failing to prevent, or bearing witness 2. to acts that transgress [the soldiers] deeply held moral beliefs and expectations [that] 3. may be deleterious in the long-term, emotionally, psychologically, behaviorally, spiritually, and socially."

Figure 2

For these reasons, I have referred to these definitions previously as first and second wave understandings of moral injury, respectively.[10] There is a shift in the Litz definition to a broader understanding, one that is not focused on the context of the military hierarchy, and one that focuses on psychological research norms. Shay, on the other hand, draws a great deal from classics and the humanities in his methodology, and also underscores the importance of institutional context and power relations. Over the past few years, these definitions have come closer together. Shay has acknowledged Litz and his coauthor's definitions as another approach to moral injury, one that, in his words, assumes "the violator [of what's right] is the self," while still others have started to use the terminology of perceived moral injury by self and moral injury by others.[11] Even so, this division can be helpful when discussing moral injury, as I will demonstrate, as it helps bring out some of the assumptions and elisions in current moral injury discourse and research.

The individualization of moral injury

There is a problem with moral injury definitions that follow the second wave, however. That problem is a focus on the individual as both the location and the source of moral injury. In most of the literature, moral injury occurs when a soldier or individual violates their own values. The commissioner and object of the injury is the soldier, the individual. The definition above by Litz and his co-authors, although helpful in many ways, does not privilege other factors or other sources that share in the responsibility for the injury. Over the intervening years, this has become more nuanced, but there is still a significant individualistic element to such definitions.

Indeed, even later definitions that attempt to de-pathologize the experience of moral injury can end up in the same conceptual place. Farnsworth et al., for example, see moral injury as "expanded social, psychological, and spiritual suffering stemming from costly or unworkable attempts to manage, control, or cope with the experience of moral pain."[12] For the authors, moral pain is natural, even potentially positive. It is a normal part of life to experience moral pain. The injury comes when one is unable to deal appropriately and in a healthy manner with that pain. Although the authors do important work by highlighting that not all suffering that we could call "moral" is pathological, the inability to cope with such pain, and so the creation of pathological suffering, seems again to fall on the agency of the individual sufferer. Indeed, the discussion of moral pain becoming moral injury reflects medical diagnosis frameworks that look at disease as either acute or chronic. There is little critical reflection, however, on such a framework and whether or not it should be applied to injuries that are best described as moral or even spiritual.

This is important, because the contexts within which moral injury occurs, either in the warzone or, if we are to extend it, within healthcare contexts, are complex. One's everyday life within military or healthcare institutions, though different in many respects, is still embedded within hierarchies, managerial and staff structures, and informed by norms, policies, and precedents over which the individual may have very little or no control. One is not always in charge, and perhaps, one is rarely so. The sense of goodness, of right and wrong, that not only comes from one's upbringing but also from the professional values one has internalized in becoming a nurse, a doctor, a chaplain, or a soldier, are not always prioritized by leadership, or by official policies. One's own values or moral worldview can come up against other values, such as the ongoing health of the organization, or in war, the overall strategy to victory. Although hospitals are not warzones, even when we compare them metaphorically, a shared tension exists between the moral striving of individuals and the ongoing needs and politics of the institution. And although hospitals not found in warzones may never or rarely encounter the conditions of war, they are still institutions that deal in matters of life and death where stakes can be quite high.

Moral Injury and Moral Distress

Helpfully, these issues of institutional culture, management structure and style, and even politics, are addressed in certain understandings of moral injury. Shay, for example, looked at the experience of veterans and saw a running theme of betrayal. Indeed, one of the main characteristics of the soldier's experience of Vietnam, one brought to the fore through both memoir and fiction over the last several decades, has been the enlisted soldier's feeling of betrayal by officers who were more concerned with their careers or their own safety over that of their soldiers, or of leaders who put them in positions where they had to actively participate in betraying their own sense of right and wrong. Shay observed this feeling of betrayal and how it ate away at the soldiers' sense of their own moral self. For Shay, it was this very relationship between leaders and subalterns within the chain of command that made such injury possible.

Moral injury, then, may be located in the soldier, but it arises from a broken relationship between superior and subordinate within the specific institutional context of the military chain of command.

Discourses in healthcare can help emphasize the institutional sources and context for moral harms. In nursing and healthcare ethics, the language developed to articulate this experience has focused on moral distress and moral residue. At least originally, moral distress was somewhat of a critique of bioethics, broadening the understanding of moral challenge and harm beyond what was seen as bioethics' singular focus on moral dilemma in discussing moral challenges in the workplace.[13] At least in its original definition, moral distress looked at the way in which nurses, in particular, may already know what the right course of action is, but cannot carry it out because of the needs of the healthcare institutions themselves, poor communication or management leadership, inadequate resources or training, or the politics of the institution.[14] If this continued and had a lasting effect, if could be called moral residue. The emphasis, then, was generally not just the difficulty of moral discernment. Instead, the point of such discourse was to articulate the difficulty of being a moral agent within a professional, institutional context, and specifically, how working in healthcare can create situations where one's sense of right and wrong comes into conflict with what the workplace requires.[15]

Similar to Shay's first wave understanding of moral injury, the moral distress literature focuses on specific healthcare sites and potentially distressing situations that can arise within those contexts. The sources of moral distress may vary, of course. Epstein and Delgado, in their overview of the literature, give several sources for such distress, including:

- Continued life support even though it is not in the best interest of the patient
- Inadequate communication about end-of-life care between providers and patients and families
- Inappropriate use of healthcare resources
- Inadequate staffing or staff who are not adequately trained to provide the required care
- Inadequate pain relief provided to patients
- False hope given to patients and families.[16]

As helpful as Shay's work and the work on moral distress can be for moving discourses of moral harm away from overly individualist methodologies, there are relationships and contexts that such approaches still do not include, at least in their formal definitions. If we are to think about the individual as embedded in various moral ecologies and institutional contexts, we can think then of concentric circles around the person. At the center is the individual, who comes to the attention of clinicians and ethicists as a sufferer in need of therapy. Around them is their home life, as well as their work life, which the previous approaches account for. If we broaden our picture, however, we see circles that are unaddressed, such as the larger social institutions, structures, and relationships in which, and through which, one's personal, family, and work life takes place. The literature discussed overly focuses, then, on the person or the person as part of a larger ecology of their immediate institutional affiliation. The rest of one's community, even society, which also deeply affects the individual and one's work-life context, is not taken into account and, if care is not taken, can even be elided altogether.

This is an overly simplistic schema of the relationship of individual to society, but it does help to give us a visual guide for where I want to go next. In the definition put forward by Litz and his co-authors, which has been a foundational definition in clinical psychological research, the context, either of the warzone or deployment back home, is not so much missing as assumed. Even so, very little time is spent examining or privileging the institutional context as a factor in moral injury. The focus, instead, is on the transgression that the soldier herself commits against her own moral code. This code is no doubt influenced by shared military moral codes, but this is not something taken up in the formal definition. Indeed, there is no reference to the very difficult moral situations created by being in an institution whose mission is to implement militarized foreign policy, policy decided on by others. The focus is on individual soldiers, what they did or did not do, what they saw or did not see. Other possible salient factors, such as the overall justice or injustice of the war or how perceptions of the morality of the war or its conduct could affect how the soldier understands the morality of her conduct in the war, are not privileged.

Shay, on the other hand, is a bit more complicated. On the one hand, he defines moral injury, particularly in his later work, as taking place in the context of the military hierarchy. Indeed, the cause of moral injury is laid not at the feet of the soldier and her own actions but at the feet of officers and even the culture of the hierarchy in general. It is the health, we could say, of that hierarchy, an institution that deeply effects the lives of soldiers, that is the cause of the injury, or at least is necessary to the injury, if not entirely sufficient. On the other hand, Shay also wants to cast moral injury as a timeless issue. His first book, *Achilles in Vietnam*, explores the *Illiad* as a source for understanding this new concept. This can be helpful in that soldiers can reframe their suffering as something that all soldiers, even the bravest, have faced throughout history. It can help veterans push back against the stigma that so often adheres to soldiers who suffer psychological traumas by reframing mental health disorders as on par with more heroic physical wounds. It can also help veterans feel less abnormal by reframing moral injury as an irreducible part of war. In this way it can be seen as something shared, as something soldiers throughout time have gone through, and not as the result of something unique an individual soldier has done.

At the same time, however, this move de-historicizes moral injury in a problematic way. The command hierarchy of today's military is very different from the hierarchy and culture of a fabled epic Greek myth. Although it is important to explore whether such harms as moral injury appear in other contexts, it creates a tension between the timeless, transcultural understanding of moral injury that Shay argues for and his emphasis on moral injury arising from a specific and quite modern command and control military hierarchy.

More important for my purposes here is how this transhistorical, transcultural emphasis on moral injury can unintentionally elide the specific politics that surround and penetrate any particular war or conflict. Quite rightly, there are always tensions during times of life and death between subalterns and their superiors, and Shay has an insight into how this relationship can give rise to moral injury. He does not address, however, how the specific politics of the time, and the broader trends of culture and public opinion, also factor into how soldiers and others view the justness of the overall war and strategy. How do politics—understood not only in terms of policy, but also the politics of one's society and culture—affect the ways in which soldiers understand the war, their participation in it, and whether or not what they are doing is for a just, unjust, or questionable cause?

This is particularly important for the wars being fought under what, before the Obama administration, was called the "Global War on Terror." Some veterans who are arguably morally injured have pointed not just to their own actions as sources of their moral injury, nor even only the military hierarchy, as one would expect from Shay's understanding of such harms. They also argue for a culpability that the broader society shares, where society has allowed or even supported what the veterans have come to see as an unjust war. One soldier, for example, Marc Loiselle, a U.S. army platoon leader in Iraq from 2003–06, reflected on his experience during the war and subsequent occupation that it made him feel like he had become a bad person because of what he did and his participation in the war. Loiselle does not absolve himself from any sin. He confides, "The secret about combat—what not even the harshest anti-war cynic will tell you—is coming home and walking around every day feeling like you're a bad person."[17] Indeed, saying that he feels like a bad person is not only a signal of possible moral injury but also shows that he feels a keen sense of responsibility.

What is interesting is that Loiselle sees this responsibility as something that is not just his but something he shares with his society. After saying how the war was not worth the lives it cost, he then incriminates his larger culture: "We talk about the superiority of our culture, but then we invade their country and set them at each other's throats like animals."[18] One need not agree with his sentiments, or with other veterans' similar sentiments, to see the broader politics that someone like Loiselle is gesturing toward. Moral injury has a dimension that is central to Loiselle's suffering and that is not quite captured in either Shay or Litz's definitions, nor even by moral distress. Loiselle is referring to a cultural narrative where his society sees itself as better than the country they are invading, a narrative his experience contradicts. On top of the policies that made up the war, a sense of politics conditions and gives rise to his moral injury on the broader, society-wide level.

Indeed, theologian Willie James Jennings gets at this understanding of moral injury by emphasizing the importance of narratives of U.S. exceptionalism in the moral injury of veterans. He is worth quoting in full:

> America is a place intoxicated with narrative power. That narrative power has been overwhelming, not only for a public habituated in its performance, but also for generations of veterans who have been subjected to its life mangling affects. Veterans have been asked to narrate their lives inside of profound contradictions—honorable service inside of dishonorable wars, virtuous actions enmeshed in violence, national celebration and admiration coupled with constant neglect. Such contradictions only intensify once they reenter a civilian world that drowns their individual stories inside an American narrative that turns their lives into nothing more than illustrations of patriotism.[19]

Jennings emphasizes the ways in which Loiselle's culture remembers its past and how such memory helps constitute the present. For Jennings, who draws on liberative theological and ethical frameworks, a fault line emerges between the story that the country tells itself about the virtuousness of its actions and its war on the one hand, and the experience of a soldier like Loiselle, which seems to contradict that narrative, on the other. The moral injury may, as I have argued elsewhere, come from such a fissure, as a form of *poisonous knowledge* about oneself and one's country that they rather not have.[20] It may also be a factor that exacerbates the injury, especially when, as Jennings writes, veterans must return home and live within this dissonance.[21] Either way, this is an element of moral injury, one that Loiselle seems to speak to, that is not easily captured by the previous approaches to moral injury.

The COVID-19 Pandemic

Although at the time of this writing there are few works in bioethics and healthcare ethics that address the pandemic through moral injury, such literature has begun. Williams et al., for example, argue rightly that the pandemic has increased the possibility for moral distress in hospitals, which they argue can transform into moral injury. The authors acknowledge issues of racism in healthcare policy and provision in general and the larger structural constraints in which healthcare workers do their jobs. Their focus, importantly, is how people can get through the pandemic without moral injury. Advocating for "psychological first aid," they detail actions to create and promote "safety, calmness, connectedness, self-efficacy, and hope" within healthcare settings. For example, when discussing how hospitals should create a "sense of safety," they describe how this should be done in pre-pandemic times:

> Psychologists can disseminate resources to assist patients and colleagues, as well as model healthy sleep, proper nutrition, regular exercise, and stress management techniques. They can engage individuals who are struggling in brief problem-solving exercises.[22]

They also argue for mindfulness in the face of the pandemic to help instill calmness. Indeed, stress management in general is their approach for managing distress so that it does not become an injury.

The responses the authors detail seem somewhat limited, much more limited than the authors themselves would want to offer. Indeed, the pandemic has created constraints that narrow the possibility for implementing more robust interventions that aim to instill safety, calm, and community. Connectedness practices that would once have been proffered have become strained or more cumbersome, as teletechnology or Zoom are now needed to mediate connectedness. Because of the pandemic, it has become very challenging for healthcare workers to eat well, exercise, and sleep when one cannot get to a source of good food, go to the gym or even walk outside in an urban environment, sleep well when one is overworked and has internalized the crisis, or does not even have time in the midst of the crisis to pursue such practices. Mindfulness is also questionable in such situations. How will being mindful of one's situation help when such a situation for some borders on the hellish?

The problem in their response to moral injury may arise from the assumed linkage of moral injury to moral distress, where injury is an outcome of untreated or prolonged distress. This is a theoretical move that is assumed and not argued for. The authors are bringing in a concept from one institutional context into another, which requires greater attention to the possible tensions and contradictions of such a linkage, as well as greater attention to the assumptions being made and that are not clarified in the paper. The lack of such conceptualization leads to therapies that seem inadequate to the task. Moral injury, which comes from a wartime context and can involve issues of profound injustice or shame at one's participation in violence, would seem to negate the possibility of calmer contexts. It is a simplification that does not do justice to the deep moral challenges that give rise to such injury, challenges that can be similar to those healthcare professionals may also be experiencing during the high-stakes conditions of a global pandemic.

The authors do acknowledge broader cultural and even political contexts in their paper, such as racism and lack of resources, and yet do not offer suggestions on how to deal with these impacts on the environment in which healthcare workers labor during the pandemic. This is due to several reasons. The first is that during an emergency, the authors are right to focus on first aid. Care to the individual in distress is important, and you must make sure the person before you has what they need to keep functioning. The second, however, is that the moral injury literature that the authors use to define such harm privileges the individual, as previously demonstrated, as the commissioner and object of the injury. These formal definitions in the moral injury literature do not take into account the larger cultural and political contexts in which moral injuries are formed, contexts that are central to the nature of the injury in question.

For example, the authors mention the lack of resource provision as a contributor to potentially morally injurious situations, but they do not go on to mention how the ongoing debate and conflicts within and between levels of government over these issues can help give rise to the moral injury and loss of hope that some may feel. The paper also does not mention the rise in protests against social distancing measures, protests that healthcare workers have seen as affecting them and those whom they care for directly. It does not mention the rhetoric of the president of the United States, members of Congress, and local and state officials, and how such polemic can affect healthcare workers. Neither does it mention the ways in which healthcare workers can feel like they have become complicit in the policy and administrative decisions that govern life and death in a healthcare setting or even with the national policy decisions around resourcing the pandemic. Whatever budget and political decisions are made around funding, stockpiling, capacity, and defunding of rural hospitals, healthcare workers must sometimes live with providing poorer treatments than they would have otherwise given due to austerity and budget decisions. And they are the ones who must be the face of their institution to patients, witnessing the harm that such decisions, even though out of their control, can do to patients. As nurses and healthcare workers at a protest in front of the White House said, "we're tired of being treated as if we are expendable."[23]

Healthcare workers, then, can feel betrayed by administrators and managers. As Alynn Schmitt McManus, a clinical social worker in St

Louis, told the *New York Times*, the betrayal felt by healthcare workers went "beyond trauma" because they felt "overwhelmed and abandoned" by bosses who "rarely acknowledge the newly relentless demands of the job."[24] This betrayal, however, can also come from politicians, as well as the broader public. This is especially the case when the broader public protests against rules that would make the situation in hospitals in particular and society in general better, or when the public elects politicians who have underfunded institutions and provisions that could have mitigated the effects of the pandemic. Such decisions, both over the long-term and the short, can be seen as not just putting one's colleagues in danger, nor even one's patients. That can be bad enough. It can also feel like such politics and polemic are directed against the safety and flourishing of one's family. In the *New York Times*, one doctor worried about bringing COVID-19 home. When he gets ready for work, he stated that his son says, "'Daddy, be very, very careful,' and I know what he's thinking."[25]

This is an important aspect of moral injury that is related to Shay's understanding of betrayal—feeling that one has been made complicit in a wrong or injustice. If bad policies or decision-making puts someone's child in danger, it is bad enough. But when someone is made the vehicle of that harm in the process of doing their job, it is their body that is delivering the consequences of bad policy to the child. What can result is a sense of complicity in endangering the one you love, or in betraying one's patients, creating a sense both of betrayal but also of feeling one has done, or might do, the unthinkable. And as too many patients die, it may not even seem to have been worth the sacrifices made.

Moral Injury and Bioethics: Future Questions and Avenues

This, of course, is an extreme example, yet in places like New York, New

Orleans, Seattle, Los Angeles, and others, it is a real fear. A level of betrayal exists involving the broader society that even Shay, who views politics as more narrowly confined to the relationship of the soldier to the military hierarchy, does not fully consider. How, then, should we understand moral injury during a pandemic like COVID-19?

First, we should see moral injury not merely as acute moral distress becoming chronic. This runs the risk of suggesting that individuals have dealt with their distress poorly or that such injury is their fault. Such an approach does not critically reflected upon the possibility of situations where someone who takes responsibility and justice seriously *should* experience such injury. In other words, are there times when injustice is so egregious, and times when one's location within the crisis is such, that one is somehow lacking some moral capacity, is morally deficient, if some degree of injury is not felt? Although unwanted and harmful, can moral injury be the sign of a praiseworthy character and moral seriousness? May it even illustrate something about character, and moral subjectivity, namely, that character makes one vulnerable to such injury precisely because one takes responsibility, justice, and the moral life seriously? Are there different forms of moral injury? And are those morally injured—or at least, those who experience some forms of moral injury—seeing something about one's society, one's culture and politics, that others cannot?

When we look at the larger cultural and political context, we can see that in the pandemic, matters not just of psychological health but of justice and social justice are profound aspects of the crisis, and of the experience of healthcare workers within the crisis. Indeed, the United States quickly became the epicenter of the crisis not simply because it was a global pandemic but also, and importantly, because of political decisions regarding preparedness, healthcare policy, healthcare funding and financing, and the ongoing battle over the nature of health insurance. This situation was exacerbated by the way in which government leadership responded to the crisis as it unfolded. Someone who takes responsibility and justice seriously cannot help but feel deeply at this situation and its political dimensions. Such deep feeling and moral seriousness, then, may not only be what we want in our neighbors, but also may be inherent in the moral life. Understanding the moral self and moral injury this way may help clinicians, chaplains, and even neighbors be more attentive to those whose strength of character may make them seem stronger or even more ethically self-sufficient than others.

Second, then, this possibility rests better if we see moral injury as something other than a diagnosis.[26] Since Litz and his co-authors published their seminal article in 2009, a number of scales and tests have appeared that attempt to diagnose moral injury, as well as various therapeutic strategies to create healing.[27] It is unclear, however, whether any diagnostic scale or survey is sufficient for a form of harm that is not psychological but moral or even spiritual. After all, we are speaking here of very subjective experiences. No objective set of principles or code applies to all that is transgressed. The overall literature assumes that it is one's own values that are transgressed and that this must be felt by the injured.[28] Moral injury, then, is very subjective, and it almost seems as if one needs to come to name one's own suffering as a moral injury. Indeed, morality is such that it would be very difficult to conclude who has the authority to diagnose one's moral or spiritual state. Even with a scale or measure, we are approaching territory here where terms such as virtue and character and wisdom may be better suited than clinical language.

If we see moral injury, then, not as a diagnosis in need of a clinical intervention, we may be able to see that at least some examples of moral injury point to society being in need of repair. Therapy, I would argue, is always an important and often critical tool for any such injury. If, however, there are political dimensions to such an injury, we can perhaps see it as reflecting a real response, a visceral insight, into the conditions and injustices of one's day. And, if there is a political dimension, responses to such an injury may require actions beyond the therapeutic.

Third, then, moral injury can be seen in a more epistemological frame. Unlike PTSD, where one can actually forget the cause of the trauma or have trouble with memory, moral injury usually revolves around a quite clear memory of the cause of the suffering. One has seen or experienced things that have changed the way they see and understand themselves and the world. It is, to use a loaded term, perhaps new knowledge, even if not wanted, that can change one quite deeply. And if it involves issues of justice and injustice, of wrong and reconciliation, such moral injuries could also provide a basis for prophetic insight, as one has seen more keenly into the demands of the present moment.[29]

I do not want to say that all moral injury is like this. It is more helpful to think of various forms of moral injury with various etiologies and meanings. My attempt here has been to think through what it might mean to acknowledge a form of moral and psychological harm conditioned significantly by the political. I use political here to signify not only policy making, but also the power maneuvers between community and state leaders that affect wellbeing, and also the power maneuvers within one's culture over which narratives are hegemonic, guiding which stories will be told and acknowledged. In the case of the current pandemic, it is hard to see the suffering and deaths without also acknowledging how deeply the crisis has been shaped by the culture wars, policies, and politics of the United States, both locally and nationally. Moral injury that results from the pandemic, then, will to some extent also be a political injury, where one has been harmed not only through the spread of a virus but how that spread and our reactions to it were formed through discourses and practices of power.

Moral injury, then, has the potential to provide some prophetic insight into the pandemic and even one's society. Such an injury can arise in many ways. If we take seriously how politics shapes such an injury, the injured have experienced the effects of such politics. They have a unique relationship to those politics, and could serve as a prophetic voice, critically informed by the ways in which the political has affected the lives of patients, healthcare workers, and communities.

Repair, then, would require not only therapeutic interventions but also political engagement in many ways. My other writings show ways that soldiers and veterans have undertaken such engagement, ranging from educating the public to direct activism. Such work usually occurs after one's military service is over, since such activism, even minimally, is quickly and easily curtailed through the military hierarchy. Something similar exists for healthcare workers during a pandemic, as so much of their time and energy is involved in caring for patients, families, and colleagues. There is little time to do much else.

Exceptions do exist. Healthcare workers in several states conducted counter-protests against groups calling for a lifting of social distancing and stay-at-home advisories, such as the "closing" of businesses. In Phoenix, Arizona, nurses stood on the steps in their scrubs, hands folded and masks on, and socially distancing, in contradistinction to the protestors who neither had masks nor were distancing safely. This also occurred in Colorado, where healthcare workers, also in scrubs, masks, and socially distancing, stood at an intersection to counter protest in the state capital. These examples reveal nurses pushing back against certain narratives of the COVID-19 pandemic as a conspiracy and trying to educate protestors and onlookers about the seriousness of what healthcare workers are doing.

Indeed, healthcare workers may need to find ways to live out their injuries in the future. Many veterans do not become aware of a moral injury until they return home. Veterans may have changed because of their experience, and those back home may not understand what they experienced and may want the veterans to pick up where they left off. They lose a community of those who understand what they have gone through, a community that can provide much support. They lose the structure of the military and may have more time to reflect on what they have done, witnessed, or failed to do.

The aftermath can and will be a time when healthcare workers start to feel something like a moral injury. As Mark Rosenberg at St Joseph's Health in Paterson, New Jersey, has said, "As the pandemic intensity seems to fade, so does the adrenaline. What's left are the emotions of dealing with the trauma and stress of the many patients we cared for. . . . There is a wave of depression, letdown, true PTSD and a feeling of not caring anymore that is coming."[30] This is occurring now and will only grow in the near future, especially as more waves of COVID-19 are set to grow in the late summer, fall, and winter. The feelings of being at the whim of political pressures and decisions, and of having insights that are being ignored in the power and budgetary struggles throughout govern- ment, may require more than therapeutic interventions. It may require political responses to match the political dimensions of the pandemic. This may mean organizing and creating networks of solidarity where healthcare workers not only treat the patients in front of them but they advocate and fight for the budgets and resources that make the best of care possible.

When we think, then, of bioethics and moral injury in the time of COVID-19, we may need a political vocabulary to add to our ethical and clinical ones, using terms such as prophetic speech and knowledge, solidarity, organizing, protest, and even coercion. This will allow healthcare workers not just to treat their personal feelings of shame, anger, guilt, and betrayal, but also feel an empowerment to change the conditions that gave rise to such injury.

Notes

1. Indeed, initial research suggests that one's political orientation signifi-
    cantly influences one's beliefs about COVID-19 and the pandemic. See for
    example, Christos A. Makridis and Jonathan T. Rothwell, "The Real Cost
    of Political Polarization: Evidence from the COVID-19 Pandemic," Social
    Science Research Network, October 29, 2020, https://dx.doi.org/10.2139/
    ssrn.3638373.

2. Joseph Wiinikka-Lydon, "Moral Injury as Inherent Political Critique: The
    Prophetic Possibilities of a New Term," Political Theology 18, no. 3 (2017):
    27; Tine Molendijk, "The Role of Political Practices in Moral Injury: A
    Study of Afghanistan Veterans," Political Psychology 40, no. 2 (2019):
    261–75; Kenneth MacLeish, "How To Feel About War: On the Politics of
    Military Psyches in the Age of Counterinsurgency," Biosocieties 14, no. 2
    (2018): 272–99.

3. Jonathan Shay, Achilles in Vietnam: Combat Trauma and the Undoing of
    Character (New York: Scribner, 1994).

4. American Psychiatric Association, Diagnostic and Statistical Manual of
    Mental Disorders, 5th Edition: DSM-5 (Washington, DC: American Psychi-
    atric Publishing, 2013), 194, 271–72.

5. See Brett T. Litz et al., Adaptive Disclosure: A New Treatment for Military
    Trauma, Loss, and Moral Injury (New York: Guilford Publications, 2015).
    Such characterological language is found at the beginning of the concept's
    history. This can be seen in the subtitle of Shay's first book on the subject,
    Achilles in Vietnam: Combat Trauma and the Undoing of Character.

6. Timothy J. Hodgson and Lindsay B. Carey, "Moral Injury and Definitional
    Clarity: Betrayal, Spirituality and the Role of Chaplains," Journal of Reli-
    gious Health 56 (2017): 1212–28.

7. Jonathan Shay, "Moral Injury," Psychoanalytic Psychology 31, no. 2
    (2014): 182.

8. Brett T. Litz et al., "Moral Injury and Moral Repair in War Veterans: A
    Preliminary Model and Intervention Strategy," Clinical Psychology Review
    29, no. 8 (2009): 695.

9. This addition to the causes of moral injury also muddies distinctions
    between PTSD and moral injury and potentially makes the concept overly
    broad. More critical attention to this claimed cause of moral injury is need-
    ed.

10. See Joseph Wiinikka-Lydon, "Mapping Moral Injury: Comparing Dis-
    courses of Moral Harm," The Journal of Medicine and Philosophy: A
    Forum for Bioethics and Philosophy of Medicine 44, no. 2 (2019): 175–91;
    Joseph Wiinikka-Lydon, Moral Injury and the Promise of Virtue (New

York: Palgrave, 2019).

11. Jonathan Shay, "Casualties," Daedalus 140, no. 3 (2011): 183; Nathan R. Stein et al., "A Scheme for Categorizing Traumatic Military Events," Behavior Modification 36, no. 6 (2012): 787, 802.

12. Jacob K. Farnsworth et al., "A Functional Approach to Understanding and Treating Military-Related Moral Injury," Journal of Contextual Behavioral Science 6, no. 4 (2017): 392.

13. This is formally similar to the origins of moral injury, which arose as a critique of PTSD, and in particular of PTSD not being able to capture the moral and spiritual dimensions of wartime mental harm.

14. See the seminal definition in Andrew Jameton, Nursing Practice: The Ethical Issues (Englewood Cliffs, NJ: Prentice-Hall, 1984).

15. Elizabeth G. Epstein and Sarah Delgado, "Understanding and Addressing Moral Distress," The Online Journal of Issues in Nursing 15, no. 3 (2010), https://www.doi.org/10.3912/OJIN.Vol15No03Man01.

16. Epstein and Delgado, "Understanding and Addressing Moral Distress."

17. Loiselle's comments were recorded in a CNN online article by Daphne Sashin titled "In Their Own Words: 8 Lives Changed by the Iraq War," CNN, December 15, 2011, https://www.cnn.com/2011/12/15/world/meast/iraq-ireporter-stories/index.html.

18. Sashin, "In Their Own Words."

19. Willie James Jennings, "War Bodies: Remembering Bodies in a Time of War," in Post-Traumatic Public Theology, ed. Stephanie N. Arel and Shelly Rambo (New York: Palgrave, 2016), 27.

20. Wiinikka-Lydon, "Moral Injury as Inherent Political Critique," 27.

21. The importance of returning home to moral injury is also something underscored by Shay. See Jonathan Shay, Odysseus in America: Combat Trauma and the Trials of Homecoming (New York: Simon and Schuster, 2010). See also Shay, "Causalities," 181.

22. Roger D. Williams, Jessica A. Brundage, and Erin B. Williams, "Moral Injury in Times of COVID-19," Journal of Health Service Psychology (May 2, 2020): 1–5 (advanced online edition).

23. Bridget Read, "'We're Tired of Being Treated as If We Are Expendable,'" The Cut, April 21, 2020, https://www.thecut.com/2020/04/nurses-coronavirus-protests-lawsuits-protective-equipment.html.

24. Jan Hoffman, "'I Can't Turn My Brain Off': PTSD and Burnout Threaten Medical Workers," The New York Times, May 16, 2020 https://www.nytimes.com/2020/05/16/health/coronavirus-ptsd-medical-workers.html.

25. Hoffman, "'I Can't Turn My Brain Off.'"

26. For another argument against moral injury as a diagnosis, see Kent D. Drescher, Jason A. Nieuwsma, and J. Swales Swales, "Morality and Moral Injury: Insights from Theology and Health Science," Reflective Practice: Formation and Supervision in Ministry 33 (2013): 50–61.

27. For information on the development and evaluation of a scale for moral injury, see Currier, Joseph M., Jacob K. Farnsworth, Kent D. Drescher, Ryon C. McDermott, Brook M. Sims, and David L. Albright. "Development and Evaluation of the Expressions of Moral Injury Scale-Military Version." Clinical Psychology & Psychotherapy 25, no. 3 (May 2018): 474–88; Nash, William P., Teresa L. Marino Carper, Mary Alice Mills, Teresa Au, Abigail Goldsmith, and Brett T. Litz. "Psychometric Evaluation of the Moral Injury Events Scale." Military Medicine 178, no. 6 (June 2013): 646–52. https://doi.org/10.7205/MILMED-D-13-00017.

28. For approaches to healing moral injury, two important developments include, first, adaptive disclosure: Litz et al., Adaptive Disclosure. A second includes prolonged exposure therapy Smith, Erin R., Jeanne M. Duax, and Sheila A. M. Rauch. "Perceived Perpetration During Traumatic Events: Clinical Suggestions From Experts in Prolonged Exposure Therapy." Cognitive and Behavioral Practice 20, no. 4 (2013): 461–70. https://doi.org/10.1016/j.cbpra.2012.12.002. See the following, which is a response to Smith et al. by those arguing for adaptive disclosure: Steenkamp, Maria M., William P. Nash, Leslie Lebowitz, and Brett T. Litz. "How Best to Treat Deployment-Related Guilt and Shame: Commentary on Smith, Duax, and Rauch (2013)." Cognitive and Behavioral Practice, Collaborative Empiricism in Cognitive Behavior Therapy, 20, no. 4 (November 2013): 471–75. https://doi.org/10.1016/j.cbpra.2013.05.002. See also Keenan, Melinda J., Vicki A. Lumley, and Robert B. Schneider. "A Group Therapy Approach to Treating Combat Posttraumatic Stress Disorder: Interpersonal Reconnection through Letter Writing." Psychotherapy (Chicago, Ill.) 51, no. 4 (December 2014): 546–54. https://doi.org/10.1037/a0036025. Farnsworth, Jacob, Kent D. Drescher, Wyatt Evans, and Robyn D. Walser. "A Functional Approach to Understanding and Treating Military-Related Moral Injury." Journal of Contextual Behavioral Science 6, no. 4 (2017): 391–97. Kristine Burkman, Natalie Purcell, and Shira Maguen, "Provider perspectives on a novel moral injury treatment for veterans: Initial assessment of acceptability and feasibility of the Impact of Killing treatment materials," Journal of Clinical Psychology 75 (2019): 79-94.

29. This may seem like an obvious statement, yet in philosophical works dealing with dignity harms, there are some arguments that such harms do not have to be felt by those harmed (Wiinikka-Lydon, "Mapping Moral Injury," 182). Such harms are also called "moral injuries," but come from a separate source than psychological approaches to moral injury discussed in these pages. For a discussion of these modes of moral injury and their

COVID-19 PANDEMIC: THE KENYAN FRONTLINER'S EXPERIENCE

SIMIYU BRAMWEL WEKESA
MBCHB, MA BIOETHICS

I am Dr. Simiyu Bramwel Wekesa, a Senior Family Medicine Resident from Kabarak University attached to AIC Kijabe Hospital for my clinical coursework. I have a Master of Arts degree in Bioethics from Trinity International University, Illinois, USA, and I have special interests in medical ethics and policy.

I consider it a privilege to share with you our experiences and ethical challenges as we take care of our patients during this COVID-19 pandemic at Kijabe Mission Hospital, Kenya. It is a level 6 B category (tertiary referral and teaching hospital) with a 365-bed capacity. When COVID-19 was declared a pandemic, we converted 80 of these beds to specifically care for COVID-19 patients. We have had an average of 5–9 suspected cases per week in the respiratory isolation (COVID-19) ward and our turnaround time for a COVID-19 test is at least one week.

Once COVID-19 was noted to be on the African continent, Kenya took a strict approach to contain the spread of the virus after its first case on March 12, 2020. This was achieved through various measures such as suspension of local and international air travel as well as limiting local travel through internal lockdown measures, both intra- and inter-country and especially in the hotspot areas, and a dusk to dawn curfew.[1] Elaborate campaigns on wearing masks in public places for all people, hand washing with soap and water and/or sanitizing, as well as physical distancing were promoted and emphasized by the Kenyan Ministry of Health. Closure of schools, restaurants, bars, and places of worship, strict public transport measures (i.e., carrying half capacity), etc. were instituted. At the same time, there was targeted screening and quarantine of infected or suspected individuals. These measures bore some fruit, as the spread of the virus has seemingly been slow.

At Kijabe hospital, an infection prevention control (IPC) team specifically for the COVID-19 pandemic was instituted to develop protocols and offer guidance on management. Measures proposed included ensuring that all patients and staff are screened before entering the hospital, taking a quick history of symptoms (cough, difficulty in breathing, fever), tracking travel or contact with possible COVID-19 cases, and measuring oxygen saturation and temperature for all coming to the hospital. Suspected outpatient cases are seen at a separate location in the hospital and sometimes consultation is done remotely (via phone). The suspected COVID-19 inpatient cases are managed in the isolation COVID-19 ward, and there are preventive measures instituted in the ward to deter the spread of the infection from patient to patient, patient to staff, or vice versa.

Lack of a known effective treatment and/or vaccination made management of the novel COVID-19 coronavirus difficult worldwide. Its novelty meant a search to understand its pathophysiology, natural course, management, complications, and preventive measures, among others. This presents some challenges to the ethics and the practice of medicine at an individual clinician, institutional, national, and global level. Nevertheless, a lot has been put together towards this thanks to many who have and continue to contribute to the wealth of knowledge about COVID-19.

After much preparation and anticipation as a hospital, we finally got our first COVID-19 positive case (this was our 27th highly suspected inpatient care COVID-19 test) about three months after the first case was confirmed in Kenya. I happened to be part of the team that took care of this patient. Mr. X presented on a Monday for a general surgery clinic follow-up for possible colostomy closure, and after review, a date was booked and he was discharged. That Thursday he presented to our Emergency Room (ER) with generalized abdominal pain, fast breathing, and was noted to be hypoxic with a high random blood sugar. Initially he was thought to have Diabetic Ketoacidosis (only), but upon thorough evaluation he was noted to have typical radiological features of COVID-19, so he was isolated and all supportive care offered to him in the COVID-19 ward's High Dependency Unit. Despite care, he continued to deteriorate within 24 hours of admission and he later coded; we did cardiopulmonary resuscitation (CPR) with intubation but sadly he died. With our turnaround time for his COVID-19 test of 6 days, we were unsure of risk, but we had handled him with some personal protective equipment (PPE). This was indeed a true test to our "preparedness" as individuals and as a hospital. Many of our healthcare workers entered quarantine as a result of caring for this patient, but luckily, no one became symptomatic.

I will attempt to represent the plight of many Kenyan, and perhaps African, healthcare workers, and the ethical challenges encountered while caring for patients during this pandemic:

1. Fear

Most healthcare workers, myself included, feared and still do fear COVID-19: the fear of being infected and dying from the virus is real. There is full awareness that we are not immune to it. This is informed by the media and published reports of healthcare workers who have been infected and many who have died in the line of duty around the world. In Africa most of the dying are young (> 60% are below 65 years of age) and so even being a young healthcare worker is not an absolute insurance against death.[2] The concern of being infected and then infecting colleagues, or worse, taking it home to your loved ones, has in a way influenced the way we practice medicine. There is a palpable need to self-protect before caring for a patient, which may suggest a deviation from the expected quality of care being offered to patients.

With the exception of those at high risk for severe forms of the disease as shown by global statistics, everyone else was expected to continue working in their various departments. However, working in the COVID-19 isolation outpatient and inpatient departments was initially voluntary but is now staffed on a rotation basis such that most if not all other department staff must cover the COVID-19 ward to minimize stigma among colleagues. If one gets sick, the hospital offers both home (house) quarantine and treatment free of charge to encourage staff to continue working. To minimize taking the infection home, there is a plan to give hospital scrubs that are worn, laundered, and left in the hospital as well as a hot shower point for all involved in patient care. Every staff member was initially given a cloth mask, but once we got our first confirmed case, everyone now gets a surgical mask. Those attending to the isolated patients get an N95 mask and other PPE. Despite these measures, there is still that inner personal debate between requiring the hospital (as the employer) to offer us protection before asking us to work and the inner desire as Christians to offer compassionate care to all who come to us, which raises the question: How best should we uphold the Hippocratic oath, Nightingale pledge, etc. in the midst of a serious infection that poses a threat to our very own lives? And how is fear affecting our clinical judgement as we care for COVID-19 patients and the other patients with unknown status?

2. Uncertainty

Being unsure of many aspects of this disease means unpreparedness at all levels of prevention and treatment even when we feel prepared. A cure or a vaccine is still elusive as of this writing, but there is hope, as a lot of research is ongoing worldwide. Our hospital infection prevention committee came up with an approach to COVID-19 care based on the Kenyan Ministry of Health (MOH), World Health Organization (WHO) guidelines, Centre for Disease Control and Prevention (CDC), CDC Africa, webinars, and other available published data from around the world. Best case scenario discussions were not uncommon. Generally, there was very little evidence to base care on at the beginning, but as evidence emerges regular reviews and updates to protocols are done. There was also a challenge accessing most of the much-needed resources at the beginning, but this is better now. Nevertheless, in our resource-limited setting, anxiety is real, and the feelings of unpreparedness and incapacity made many healthcare workers wonder what would happen if many of them got sick too, let alone their patients. There has been a lot of change in what seems to be the effective normal standard supportive care but then after further scrutiny seems not to work for COVID-19. At such times of uncertainty there is some likelihood that harm is inevitably caused even as we try to treat this mysterious disease (an enigma indeed) as evidenced by the regular protocol updates/changes and newer practice recommendations globally. Amidst such uncertainty in the practice of medicine, how can the goals of medicine still be ethically achieved?

3. Physician-Patient Relationship

The special physician-patient relationship is based on trust, and it requires every physician to put the patient's welfare first before the physician's (self) interest. COVID-19 has attacked this trust in many ways. Trust is earned through the communication of the intentions and the actions of the involved parties, but COVID-19 poses a challenge to this because of the changes introduced in some actions as well as the intentions. Self-preservation as a human instinctual reaction is inevitable at such a time. Medical consultations while wearing a face mask and other PPE creates an "invisible" but real distance between the physician and the patient. Practically, physical distancing means that the patient sits further from the doctor in the consultation room than before. There is minimal contact with the patient and sometimes no physical examination, which further increases that distance. Some medical consultations are done over the phone and patients are discharged home with medication without physically meeting a physician. The consultation room doors are sometimes kept open (an infection prevention measure), but this affects the patient's privacy. Most patients have actually voiced feeling distant from their healthcare providers, and some in the isolation ward feel very lonely. Some have even reported that the quality of care has been reduced. Some patients were reluctant to disclose travel or relevant COVID-19 history for fear of isolation and/or being subjected to a perceived lower quality of care in the isolation ward or quarantine.

Again, once isolated as a suspected case, patient confidentiality is generally not protected since there are many people who are interested in the patient's information and test results, including the clinical and non-clinical hospital staff, family, friends, and neighbors too. A confidentiality breach is more likely detrimental to the physician-patient relationship than not. Inasmuch as there is a lot of good effort in care, this pandemic has in different ways affected the trust that is the cornerstone of the physician-patient relationship. How can we best maintain trust in the physician-patient relationship during a crisis like COVID-19?

4. Harm

It is important to be aware of the various ways in which harm to both patients and healthcare workers can occur during this COVID-19 pandemic in order to curtail its effects on healthcare provision. Avoiding harm in healthcare emanates from the ethical principle of nonmaleficence. Here are some of the ways in which harm towards patients and healthcare workers can occur during COVID-19.

Psychological harm: The fear of COVID-19 infection and death have caused significant stress and anxiety to both patients and staff. The treatment of COVID-19 patients in isolation from other patients and quarantine worsens their psychological stress. Diminished focus on psychosocial and spiritual wellbeing has caused a negative impact on the patients in the isolation ward. Isolation is a scientifically proven infection control measure, but it brings with it some challenges. Isolation means minimal contact or interaction with healthcare workers and no hospital visitation by relatives (often in Africa when one is unwell, his/her family, friends, neighbors, church members—you name it—would try and visit their loved one in the hospital, but not so during COVID-19 times), and this has left many patients feeling abandoned. Handshakes or hugs and other forms of appropriate touch are an essential component of African culture as a way of human connection. With this in mind then, the necessary physical distancing has in a way caused social distancing in Africa. But it is better to be alive and well rather than die holding on to culture. Perhaps COVID-19 is pointing us towards a universal culture as human beings.

Medical care associated harm: Protocols for COVID-19 management took days and months to develop, and since its emergence as an outbreak, then an epidemic, and now a pandemic, there have been multiple reviews and revisions to those protocols based on the available evidence, experiences, and expert opinions from different parts of the world. As such, the quality of care keeps improving, but that also may imply that those who were cared for before did not receive the best and that some may have received harmful treatments. Currently, there is commendable sharing of available and emerging evidence regarding this disease, but that does not always guarantee that it reaches all intended users on time. The need to quickly mobilize human resources in such times means people have to quickly acquire and apply new knowledge far from their daily practice to assist in care of surging numbers of patients. This is in many ways helpful, but at the same time healthcare workers have to offer what they are not necessarily good at, and harm may possibly occur. Delays in care have occurred due to the time taken to don and doff PPE during emergencies, especially when short-staffed, and sometimes a total lack of PPE may mean no care.

Stigma: "A special harm." Suspected and confirmed COVID-19 patients need to be isolated, and all identified contacts for the confirmed cases are required to be quarantined as well. For fear of being infected both suspected and confirmed staff and patients are shunned by colleagues, friends, and relatives at home, at their work places, and even on public transport (our staff have reported being shunned on public transport when donning their hospital uniform, their neighbors do not interact with them as usual, and even their children cannot play with their friends freely in the neighborhoods). Stigma causes discrimination, which in turn leads to injustice. Stigma is injustice being meted upon COVID-19 suspected or confirmed patients and healthcare workers. As a hospital, we are working on measures to mitigate this stigma among healthcare workers and in the community.

Just allocation of scarce resources: The ethical principle of justice required us to have clear guidelines on whom to intubate and resuscitate and whom not to. Such selection means that some patients get comfort care, and we allow inevitable death to happen, while others are treated aggressively to avert avoidable death. Upon careful evaluation at admission, those who required mechanical ventilation and met our set criteria were intubated on a first come first served basis; for those who did not meet the criteria or when our capacity was full, we referred them to the nearest government or private hospital. Making those decisions was difficult for most of us. Healthcare workers are trained to save lives and to not allow death. Allowing inevitable death, I believe, is hardest in our African setting, and this is causing moral distress and/or injury to the healthcare workers' conscience. There is a national psychological counselling program free of charge for all healthcare workers. Our hospital has its own virtual and physical psychological counselling program and chaplaincy services for staff to help them deal with moral trauma. Also, how fair is it to allocate most of our available resources, both material and human, towards COVID-19 as compared to other health conditions? The closure or downscaling of scheduled clinics or checkups, immunization and nutrition services, antenatal clinic and community outreach services, among others—all done as infection prevention measures but also meant to allow available resources to focus on COVID-19 care—might eventually result in the emergence of previously eliminated communicable diseases, and poor control of non-communicable chronic conditions due to poor follow up. Countrywide, the usual number of patients in the hospitals has generally reduced and the fear of this repercussion is real and expected in the coming months.

All in all, there are a lot of achievements to be grateful for both now and in the near future. At Kijabe Hospital, we appreciate the multidisciplinary team approach in protocol development and implementation. PPE availability has markedly improved. There is rotation of staff working in the COVID-19 ward to reduce stigma. Psychological counselling and chaplaincy services are available to all affected staff (and patients) to ensure mental and spiritual sanity even as we take care of patients. Free testing and treatment are offered to infected and affected staff as per our protocol. The hospital staff who are at high risk of infection and face worse prognoses according to global statistics are exempted from direct clinical work. An 80-bed capacity hospital wing for COVID-19 patients is available; it is bigger and better than most government facilities currently around the country, both from infrastructure and human resource standpoints. Our rigorous screening of all who come to the hospital for care helps protect staff and other patients from infection. As a country (Kenya) we have managed to keep the infection rates low, although now cases are rising as we are able to test more people. Our healthcare system is not overwhelmed yet, and this has allowed continued efforts to increase capacity around the country. The current health infrastructure and human resource boost will hopefully be beneficial beyond this COVID-19 pandemic. Healthcare is now noticeably a priority for our government and hopefully going forward we will see more funding in this sector.

In conclusion, COVID-19 is a mysterious disease that has posed both medical and ethical challenges to us at Kijabe hospital. Globally, it has caused a shift in the normal practice of medicine, as well as a cultural shift in human interactions. The resultant consequences are yet to be fully understood as the pandemic is still unfolding. This requires careful scrutiny going forward.

As a final exhortation at such a time as this, we are all reminded of God's commandment to "love your neighbor as self" with the love that bears all things, believes all things, hopes all things, and endures all things (1 Cor 13: 4–8). A COVID-19 positive person may prove to be troublesome to love because of the threat to our own lives, but let us strive to love and serve them regardless. Serve them as unto the Lord for they, just like human masters, may not reward us accordingly, but our God in heaven will (Col 3:23). Let us have and share hope at this time of stress and anxiety around us, the hope in our Lord Jesus Christ. Keep safe. Do your part, for by so doing you are being a brother's keeper.

Notes

1. Ujuru Kenyatta, "Address to the Nation by H.E. Uhuru Kenyatta, C.G.H, President of the Republic of Kenya and Commander-in-Chief of the Defence Forces on COVID-19, Commonly Known as Coronavirus at Harambee House, Nairobi on 15th March 2020," president.go.ke, March 15, 2020, https://www.president.go.ke/2020/03/15/address-to-the-nation-by-h-e-uhuru-kenyatta-c-g-h-president-of-the-republic-of-kenya-and-commander-in-chief-of-the-defence-forces-on-covid-19-commonly-known-as-coronavirus/.

2. Keith P. Slugman et al., Younger Ages at Risk of Covid-19 Mortality in Communities of Color," Gates Open Research 4, no. 69 (2020): https://doi.org/10.12688/gatesopenres.13151.1.

THE *IMAGO DEI* AND THE INFINITE VALUE OF HUMAN LIFE

MATTHEW LEE ANDERSON, DPHIL

I. Introduction

America's response to COVID-19 has brought substantive questions about how we value human life to the surface of our public consciousness. In both social and medical contexts, we have been confronted by the challenge of determining the lengths to which it is reasonable to go in order to save or extend human lives. Communities have closed down public commerce, sending millions of workers home and expanding food insecurity.[1] Long term care facilities were barricaded to attempt to prevent exposure to vulnerable people.[2] Prisons were isolated, while nursing homes effectively became prisons.[3] Hospitals also imposed restrictions on caretakers for those under their care: complaints about families having to FaceTime their hospital-bound loved-ones proliferated through social media.[4]

Such restrictive policies quickly generated a counterreaction, which challenged the premise that going to such lengths to contain COVID-19 was worth the collateral damage being imposed. Responsible critics noted that enforced social distancing generated massive economic devastation, which has historically been correlated with rising mortality rates and which disproportionately affects working-class Americans.[5] They also raised concerns that both voluntary and involuntary delays in medical care contributed to the rise in all-cause mortality, in addition to rises in suicides and drug abuse.[6]

Determining what sorts of policies we ought to adopt within a pandemic poses difficult questions for Christian ethicists. Judgments about policies' effectiveness seems to require aggregating deaths and comparing tradeoffs, forms of reasoning that seem ineradicably consequentialist or utilitarian.[7] As Rebecca Mitsos writes about visitor policies that hospitals developed in response to COVID-19 for parents of sick children:

Such policies are always developed for utilitarian reasons that sacrifice some benefits for individual patients and families to maximize benefits for the community. The community benefit accrues because such policies limit the spread of infection. During the COVID-19 pandemic, such policies also allow the conservation of scarce PPE [personal protective equipment]. But they impose burdens on parents and may be psychologically detrimental for individual patients.[8]

Not surprisingly, a number of high-profile Christians challenged the utilitarianism embedded within discussions about the value of various public policy responses by asserting that every individual is made in the image of God.[9] There are two distinct ways of framing the use of the *imago Dei* by Christians averse to utilitarianism: that the individual has "infinite value," and that his or her life cannot be aggregated and traded off against the value of other lives.

These inferences are extremely intuitive for many Christians, and conveniently supply a bulwark against a utilitarianism that would occasionally generate morally repugnant outcomes.[10] For instance, John Kilner raises concerns about employing the economically loaded language of "value" or "worth" for describing the special status of human beings, as it seems to put human beings on a scale that would require balancing lives against other goods. Eventually, the value of those other goods might outweigh the value of an individual life. While the assertion of *infinite* value seems to escape the problem, Kilner contends that such an approach risks implying "human beings rival God in their worth."[11] Practically, a commitment to the infinite value of a person's life simply seems untenable. For one, preserving the lives of infinitely valuable persons would seem to require a no-risk threshold for engaging in necessary activities, especially when there is a pandemic afoot. One might conclude that the assertion of infinite value is either empty rhetoric or requires extreme, untenable sacrifices to save a life. There are limits to the types of costs we are willing to pay in order to add more time to our own lives, or even to add to the lives of others who are dependent upon us.[12]

These threads need unraveling in order to specify what the assertion that every individual is infinitely valuable means and what ethical implications it might or might not have for our response to a pandemic. In what follows I offer a hasty sketch of the doctrine of the *imago Dei* to argue that the peculiar significance of humanity's infinite value does *not* require us to seek the infinite, or even maximum, duration for our lives and permits some comparative judgments between groups in forming public policies. These considerations are both exploratory and tentative, not to mention incomplete: the "image of God" is not so load-bearing that one can generate every norm one needs for responsible action in a pandemic from it. Yet I try to supply enough detail to the doctrine in order to see how it might inform three distinct questions: what sorts of visitation policy hospitals or nursing homes should adopt for family members during COVID-19, how we assess the success of social distancing and lockdowns, and whether we can prioritize individuals for ventilator care in triage situations.

II. The *Imago Dei* and the Value of (a) Human Life

Jesus Christ is "the image of the invisible God, the firstborn of all creation" (Col 1:15, NASV). Though theological reflection about the *imago Dei* has frequently started elsewhere, Paul's correlation of the *eikon* of the invisible God with the person of Christ is the locus from which all other reflection about the doctrine should radiate.[13] Because of the incarnation, Paul is able to peer behind Genesis 1's ascription of the *imago Dei* to humanity's original parents and see the image of God within the life of the Triune God: No one is capable of perfectly imaging God save God alone. As such, the incarnate Christ can say the previously unthinkable to Philip: "He who has seen me has seen the Father" (John 14:9). To learn what it means to be the *image of God*, then, requires beginning with the concrete, irrepeatable life of Jesus Christ.

The barest sketch of the form of Christ's life and its significance for understanding humanity must suffice. First, Christ's life is determined by his office as Savior of the world.[14] His humanity exists only within this indissoluble connection—namely, that he is the one who comes *from* and lives *for* God, and who, because his work is one of redemption, comes *from* and lives *for* humanity.[15] Christ is born from a Virgin as a real man, and he dies as one as well. In both moments we see his humanity uniquely surrounded by the empowering presence of God himself: he is conceived by the Holy Ghost and raised by the power of that same Spirit on the third day (Luke 1:35; Rom 8:11). Christ's humanity is exclusively determined by his union with the Father and the corresponding work he is sent to accomplish on our behalf. There is no one else who can fulfill this office: Christ is the only-begotten Son of God, the incarnate Lord whose irrepeatable work discloses the uniqueness of his person. Though he is surrounded by his mother and disciples on the cross, he alone is Savior of the world.

Second, this office occurs within a lifespan: Christ is born, lives, and dies.[16] As he comes from God, so he goes to him: "Into your hands I commend my spirit," he announces as he enters into death (Luke 23:46, AKJV). The duration of his life is tied to his work: only after he says "it is finished" is he free to go to the Father. Even so, Christ does not intentionally choose his own death, but yields himself up to it beneath the providential care of God: indeed, in his agony in the Garden he pleads for such a cup to be removed from him (Luke 22:42). Only from the standpoint of Christ's resurrection do we discover that this death is both a judgment on sin and our liberation from it: because Christ rises, we say that the Friday on which he died is good (1 Cor 15:17).

Finally, Christ's office as Savior is woven throughout his organic existence as an embodied human being.[17] Christ is God enfleshed: in his miracles and his teaching, he is never less than a human being whose frame is fashioned from the dust of the earth.[18] Christ's sanctified humanity is apparent even when Mary visits Elizabeth when she is pregnant with our Lord: "The true light of the world," Karl Barth writes, "shines already in the darkness of the mother's womb."[19] And when he dies, his body is laid reverently in the tomb: though he has gone into the hand of God, the disciples still revere his flesh, which is the place of God's empowering presence upon the earth. Christ's bodily powers uniquely enable him to fulfill his vocation: his organic life is the newer and better tabernacle, equipped and endowed for his work as savior and so itself deserving of honor and respect.

While Christ is the image of God, other human beings are created *in* and *according to* that image. As Kilner notes, those prepositions underscore Christ's unique status as the *imago Dei*: only Christ can say that if we have seen Him, we have seen the Father.[20] Yet to be created *in* and *according* to that image means our humanity corresponds to Christ's. We are *from* and *for* God, and we are *from* and *for* our neighbors. We can never cease to be the creatures who, alone among all God's creation, are created in and according to his image: our ordering and determination for God and our neighbor are indelible marks upon our nature, so that we could not eradicate them if we tried. Yet to be created in and according to Christ's image means we are also called with Christ to refract and magnify God's glory through the unique vocation for which we are endowed. As Kilner writes: "Creation *in* God's image is God's expressed *intention* that people evidence the special connection they have with God through a meaningful reflection of God."[21] If we are made *in* the image of God, we are responsible to also live *according to* it—conforming our own lives to that of Jesus Christ. The doctrine of the *imago Dei* means that we must respect our neighbors not only because they are oriented toward God, but because in our orientation toward God we are called to conduct ourselves in correspondence to Christ's life.

Such an account has significant implications for how we understand the value of human beings. As the image of God, Christ discloses the value of humanity in his assumption of our nature in the incarnation, through his liberation of the same in his crucifixion, and by its renewal in his resurrection. The infinite love of God for human beings is the source and grounds of our worth, and that worth is inextricable from the aim of such love, which is to bring us to our beatitude through union with God. We can and must speak of the infinite value of human life, then: but that value is constituted by our freedom to be with the eternal, infinite God as the creatures for whom God has died. It is not founded immanently within our lives as creatures, nor does it emerge out of natural capacities or aptitudes. Instead, our infinite value arises from the fact that, of all God's creatures, we are the ones who are with God in Christ's death and resurrection. The dignity of humanity is thus, as Barth, Paul Ramsey, and others have said, an "alien dignity": it falls upon us as a light from above.[22]

The infinite value of each individual is especially disclosed through our irreplaceability, along with our unique capacity to manifest the love of God to our neighbor. There is no one else who can stand for us in the matter of our union with Christ: though we are baptized in the company of witnesses, baptism confirms the work of God in us alone.[23] Being created in God's image means having this particularity: the individual is not subsumable into the value of the species, nor into any other way of aggregating human beings.[24] Nor is the vocation to which they are called able to be filled by anyone else: the peculiar set of obligations and responsibilities that are placed upon us by the contingencies of our birth mean we have a unique task.[25] No one else can fulfill our responsibility to honor our father and mother for us; no one else has our particular endowment, our bodies, which pervasively shape the way our lives bear witness to the superfluity of God's grace. This irreplaceability is not *itself* the source or basis of value: every snowflake is unique, but not especially valuable just as such. Yet the basis of our value in our relatedness to God is disclosed only within the particular organic life God has given each of us and through the distinct task he has called us to do.[26]

As with Christ, though, our irreplaceable witness to God's love happens within a definite span of time: we are born and die, a movement that is sanctified by Christ's undertaking of it. While the infinite value of human life pervades each moment of our organic existence, it is especially crystallized at our death.[27] In death we go immediately into the hand of God: though we might die surrounded by family and friends, nothing and no one stands between us and God's presence. The basis of our infinite value is, in that moment, fulfilled—while at the same time our irreplaceability as persons is crystallized, for we leave behind a gap in the world that no one else can fill. Christ's witness to the power of death sanctions resistance; his agony in the garden indicates that death must be accepted only when the providential care of God makes it clear we cannot do otherwise. That acceptance will eventually be required of us all, as Christ does not permit us to escape it outright: he has walked the path of death before us, defeating it as an enemy so that we walk the same in confidence and peace. Death, as Saint Paul writes, has lost its "sting," which allows him to employ the imagery of "sleep" for those who await the resurrection of the dead (1 Cor 15:55, 15:6). The rest and repose such imagery conveys indicate that death can be something different than our violent sundering from our loved ones: with Christ, our death can also be the culmination and completion of our vocation to bear witness to God's love.[28] Paul is explicit that he would find it better to "depart and be with Christ," but he remains on for the sake of those churches to whom he is an apostle (Phil 1:23, NASV). The race he runs has a discrete course, with a definite destination. Only when that race is concluded is he free to go to the Father. The infinite value of human life does not permit us to demand infinite duration under the domain of sin.[29]

III. The Value of Life and Thresholds of Risk

Though what I have supplied is nothing more than a sketch of the *imago Dei,* it indicates that the doctrine has a twofold ethical salience: on one side it discloses something about the person whose life is in peril—namely, that they are a person for whom God has died. On the other side, it discloses something about our responsibility as those who might rescue or benefit them—namely, that our responsibility to live according to Christ's image demands we take up our cross and serve them in the manner that he did. To think about humanity as made according to God's image does not only mean identifying the source or basis of a person's dignity; it also demands identifying those practices that would enable and allow us to conform to God's image in Jesus Christ. Christ became a man to liberate those made according to his image from the powers of sin and death, so that we might refract God's glory in and through the unrepeatable distinctness of our lives. Such a characterization is not merely aesthetic or rhetorical, but generates practical norms that become especially salient when life is threatened, as in a pandemic.

The assertion of the infinite value of a human life raises difficult questions about the lengths to which we should go in order to protect it. Such questions came to the forefront of our medical system, as many hospitals and long-term care centers restricted family members from visiting and caring for their loved ones.[30] One survey of Michigan hospitals, for instance, found that all 49 hospitals that responded changed their visitation policies: 48 of them implemented "no visitor" policies to intensive care units, 19 of which did not make any exceptions.[31] Such limitations were regarded as necessary in part because of shortages of personal protective equipment, which would have increased the possibility of exposure for both healthcare professionals, patients, and family members who visit. The risks of an infected family member exposing others within the hospital were exacerbated by America's public health response to COVID-19, which rarely involved extensive contact tracing, effective quarantines, or sufficient testing.[32] In order to compensate for such limitations, many hospitals and long-term care centers turned to video conferencing. Yet even this imposed additional tolls on staff, who faced the added stress of upset patients and family members.[33] Not surprisingly, such policies meant many people died alone—which adds a layer of trauma to the person dying, his or her family, and the staff who are responsible to care for them in their final hours.[34]

The account of the *imago Dei* I have offered here, though, provides some reason for hospitals and nursing homes to adopt a higher-than-zero risk threshold for transmitting COVID-19 and adopt more capacious family visitation policies. Few people think that death is trivial, yet the account of the *imago Dei* I have defended would entail that it is extremely weighty. What happens at the end of a life concentrates and distills the meaning of all that has come before. How we die, and how we help others die, is a focal practice for our belief in the power of the resurrection. While we all enter death alone, we hope to begin the journey surrounded by those whose lives have been most bound up with ours—our family and intimate friends. Though this journey is sometimes painless, those who make it often need aid and comfort to peacefully enter their rest. The agitation and struggle that mark our lives can be especially acute at their end; many of us need others to carry the cross that has been placed upon us all, so that we are able to "sleep" in peace. Of all the Christian work to be done in medicine, hospice care uniquely embodies the witness to our belief that every individual has infinite value in their relatedness to the risen Christ. By compassionately accompanying persons through their final days and hours, we may help them say of their death that it was "good." In so doing, both the dying and the community around them live according to the image Christ has given us in his own passion and resurrection.[35]

Such a responsibility means that it is unreasonable to adopt *zero-risk* visitation policy—especially when caretakers are themselves at a low risk of serious health complications. Many caretakers will have strong reasons to place *themselves* at risk of infection by visiting a hospital. Though some families would opt for video conferences, others will see such means of being "present" with their loved ones who are at risk of death as too limiting.[36] And for good reason. As the cessation of a person's organic existence, death's centrality to the human experience rests upon a fundamental affirmation of the value of a person's bodily life and presence with us. Though a video conversation might provide some consolation, the medium is incongruous with the nature and significance of what is transpiring, which demands touch.[37] Families would still gain closure, eventually, but the consolation of knowing one has done everything possible to ensure our loved one sleeps peacefully is harder to come by without being present in those final moments. There is thus reason to think some people would risk their health to do so. Indeed, being actively present at a loved one's death is such an important moment that there is reason to think that many people would accept a *high* risk of being infected to do so, rather than only a *low* risk. Even if they do not, having the *choice* might mitigate the trauma they feel if they decline, as they would at least be expressing their agency.

Yet the risk threshold for visitors *being infected* is distinct from the risks of *infecting others* that hospital visitors bring. If family members accept the risk of being infected, hospitals must manage the risk of them infecting others. Yet the infinite value of human life does not permit the pursuit of infinite duration, and the presence of loved ones at the moment of death is extremely weighty. As such, it seems reasonable for hospital and long-term care centers to offer wide accommodations to family caretakers for patients in intensive care units.

Such accommodations need not be cost-free to the family members. What sorts of costs might be reasonable to impose are nebulous, and almost certainly dependent upon broader prudential considerations about levels of compliance with broader public health directives, available resources for contact tracing, and so on. We might imagine, though, requiring family members to quarantine for two weeks after the visit, as their exposure would put them at significant risk of unknowingly infecting others.[38] If healthcare resources are scarce and communities wanted to further dissuade visitors, they might also impose costs on family members by moving them to the back of the line for ventilation, should they fall ill and require acute care. This type of cost would be extreme, but might be reasonable if PPE were also unavailable, as the risks of be-ing infected while visiting would be much higher than they might be otherwise. In areas where the volume of cases threatens the integrity of the medical system, communities might attempt to hold family mem-bers who upon leaving the hospital act as vectors for the disease civilly liable, which would dissuade them from violating self-quarantine. Given such stakes, some sick patients might try to prevent their loved ones from visiting. Yet preserving the freedom for families to choose their path would honor the distinct importance of death for a person's life in a way that absolute prohibitions on visits fails to do.

Heightening the costs on family members who visit hospitals *after* they leave is crucial, as known exposure raises the probability that they will unknowingly infect others. The knowledge that one has had expo-sure to an infectious disease makes a difference to how they are obligated to act in a pandemic: if we permit individuals to hazard their own health in visiting their family members, their known exposure imposes new responsibilities on them to reduce the chances of infecting others all the way to zero, if possible. The infinite value of human life does not permit demanding infinite duration for our own lives, but it also does not entail we are free to impose unreasonable risks on others either, especially in a context where viral spread means those risks might compound expo-nentially. And clearly, the intention to not infect others when one has been knowingly exposed is insufficient on its own to make undertaking ordinary behaviors permissible. According to the doctrine of double ef-fect, the negative effects of our actions cannot be intended, but must be accepted as side-effects.[39] Intending a morally valuable end, though, is a minimal condition for determining whether our act is permissible: we must also show due regard toward those innocent individuals who our actions negatively affect. We have duties to mitigate the damage they suffer, and may even have responsibilities to rescue them afterward, if we are able. In that light, our knowledge of how probable negative side-effects are is crucial for determining whether we are licitly fulfilling our intention. The known probability of negative side-effects establishes an epistemic threshold for whether our choices satisfy the doctrine's constraints. As their likelihood seems to go up, so does our responsibility to take steps to mitigate them. If we fail to do so, we are more culpable than if we had less reason to believe they would occur. When brought into the context of a pandemic, such a position implies that having two tiers of social practice for mitigating the spread of a disease is reasonable: knowledge of exposure requires a *zero-risk* approach for further transmission, while uncertainty requires something like a *risk-mitigation* approach.

IV. Aggregations and Comparisons

Affirming the infinite value of human life is often regarded as a bulwark against utilitarian calculi, which seek to quantify, aggregate, and maximize the benefits of our choices. On the account of the image of God sketched above, the infinite value that individuals have is not indexed to their capacities or attributes. Instead, it is constituted by their unique relatedness to God, and to the irreplaceable witness to his love that their life embodies—a uniqueness and irreplaceability that are especially transparent at their death, but which subsist at every moment of their life. If such an account permits risk *mitigation* as an appropriate response to the unique challenges a pandemic poses, it also seems to sanction both certain types of aggregate judgments about the effectiveness of our policies and comparative judgments about what groups should receive resources.[40]

Honoring the irreplaceability and infinite value of each person requires seeking to prevent their premature deaths. While there is no sanction for seeking infinite duration for a life, the spread of a pathogen like SARS-CoV-2 shifts the "default" for many people's lives, or what would happen to them without any type of intervention.[41] The known spread of a disease like COVID-19 means that our policy response is a form of rescue: changes to our social policies through voluntary or imposed social-distancing or lockdowns are aimed at *preventing* people who are vulnerable from dying either earlier than they otherwise might *or* in a worse manner than they otherwise might.

Such a context has significant implications for how we weigh the success of the policies we adopt in response to a pandemic and how we identify which policies appropriately honor the individual as made in the image of God. In the first place, the affirmation of the infinite value of individuals does not obviously preclude aggregating the number of deaths "caused" by a pandemic in order to partially determine the effectiveness of our response.[42] When the United States passed 100,000 deaths attributed to COVID-19, the *New York Times* printed the (known) names of the disease's victims.[43] Listing the number of deaths aggregates the names of individuals, each of whom has an infinite value and leaves behind an irreplaceable gap. In this way, it is a unique type of aggregation, as it does not attempt to quantify the value of what is lost in ways that could establish comparative judgments *except* on the same terms (unlike "quality adjusted life years," which permits comparisons not only on the basis of the number of years saved but the criteria by which we are determining "quality").[44]

Yet the account of the image of God sketched above is also commensurate with policies that would prioritize protecting vulnerable populations, for two reasons. First, a policy ordered toward saving the most lives would require special attention to those individuals who are most at risk in order to be maximally effective. Second, as noted above, the doctrine of the image of God requires attending to the *manner* in which people die. Dying is rarely as peaceful as simply falling asleep. Yet dying from COVID-19 often involves hospitalization, requires isolation (even if family caretakers are permitted to visit), and frequently includes uncomfortable interventions like ventilation. Even if the badness of dying from COVID-19 is equivalent or marginally better than death from other causes, preventing vulnerable populations from becoming infected gives them and our health-care systems more time to ensure that they go into the hand of God surrounded by their loved ones.

This special concern for the "vulnerable" should include those who are elderly. As noted above, the infinite value of human life is present in each and every one of its moments, regardless of our capacities or consciousness: no part of the time we are given is more valuable than another, nor is any form of bodily life more valuable than another. The fact that some people are nearer the end of their life than the beginning does not mean that their deaths cannot be premature: those who age bear witness to the duration and faithfulness of God's love in a particular way, as they demand the care and support of their families and communities in a particular way. It is reasonable to see the death of an infant as more tragic than the death of those at the outer reaches of their lifespan, as we want every person to enjoy time. Yet that distinct tragedy does not entail that the badness of death for those who are over 75 can be discounted, in such a way that we would have no reason to prioritize protecting their lives in a pandemic. The priority of protecting the "vulnerable" should not discriminate on the basis of how many years they might have remaining, as the value of human life does not depend upon its (youthful) capacities and powers: The deaths of the saints are precious in God's eyes, regardless of when they occur.[45]

At the same time, the kind of comparative choices that protecting the vulnerable requires become permissible when we are trying to rescue others but have limited resources, even though they would not be licit in other contexts. Suppose you are a fireman holding a net for two people, both of whom are jumping from a burning building. If you do nothing, the "default" is that both people will die. Running to catch one will preclude catching the other, yet this is not inherently discriminatory. As both people would otherwise die without your presence, rescuing one does not disrespect the infinite value of the other. One might have reasons for a choice that would express invidious discrimination against one of them: one might *not* save a sixty-year-old African American, for instance, because one is a racist *or* because one thinks young people's lives are more valuable. But these are choices *against* a person: all-else-being-equal, a choice *for* a person when one is choosing between them does not entail a discriminatory choice *against* the other, even when one chooses for a person on the basis of a trait that the other lacks.[46]

To see this, suppose Bill is choosing to marry either Elizabeth or Claire, both of whom have upstanding character and are equally valuable. His choice of Elizabeth because she has blonde hair does not impugn the dignity of Claire because she does not. Bill may be perfectly indifferent to red hair, or even find it quite beautiful but not to his taste. That choice is very different than a case of rescue, of course, in which lives are at stake. But it indicates that in certain contexts choices for persons can be made without them being against others in a way that would be disrespectful or denigrating. Additionally, Bill's choice has this much in common with cases of rescue: it establishes a partial moral bond with Elizabeth that does not exist with Claire. This matters more for choices in rescue than we might think: a rescuer stands in a unique relationship to the one rescued, such that they are owed gratitude. An individual might choose to rescue a young person rather than an old person because they hope to enjoy the goods of friendship such a bond might establish for a longer period of time—or they might rescue an old person rather than a young one because they think that is what respect for elders demands. As long as one is not actively denigrating the other person by implying that their value is less than the value of the person saved, such choices need not be *inherently* discriminatory. Such an account generalizes to assessing policies like lockdowns, which might save lives in ways that are differentiated across a society.

However, two qualifications are necessary. First, I would stress that the permissibility of making a choice to prioritize saving group [x] and not group [y] is confined to when we have limited resources. In a situation where one is capable of saving everyone, deciding not to do so is presumptively a choice *against* that person, such that one would have to show considerable countervailing evidence to explain why it is not.[47] If it were the case that a social policy responding to the pandemic might save an equivalent number of lives (especially among vulnerable people) without contributing to a rise in unexplained all-cause mortality, that is obviously the path we should pursue. Second, such comparative choices are not *inherently* discriminatory—but they might be discriminatory *in fact*. If one lives in a context, for instance, where African Americans are routinely chosen *against*, then one faces a higher threshold for justifying one's comparative choice to save a white person rather than a black person. Similarly, if someone routinely denigrates blond-haired women, then their choice to save a red-haired woman rather than a blonde-haired woman merits a high degree of skepticism. We can even go one step further, I think, and say that a social context might require us to choose to save one group and not the other out of considerations of justice: a long social and cultural history of invidious discrimination against the elderly or disabled is sufficient to entail that one has presumptive obligations to save them—if only because one otherwise perpetuates such attitudes, even if one has otherwise acted innocently.

It is easy to see from here how this framework can be extended into questions of prioritizing treatment in ICUs when ventilators and other equipment are scarce. Honoring the infinite value of human life is compatible with an effort to save the most lives—rather than saving the highest number of quality-adjusted life years. At the same time, such a stance would not require a "first come, first served" policy, nor would it entail that those who have underlying comorbidities be pushed to the back of the line for ventilators because they might be expected to remain on one longer or have worse odds of survival. An account of the infinite value of human life does not generate a complete theory of the just distribution of health care: it does not *require* a particular way of establishing priority. But it does permit prioritizing care in order to ensure that as many people can receive it as possible. Honoring the infinite value of human life under conditions of scarcity does not require us either to expend all our resources to save a single individual, nor to throw ourselves on the blind forces of chance or fate. While the prudential choices to give a ventilator to one person and not another are fraught with danger, doing so reasonably is compatible with honoring the infinite value of individuals who are made in God's image.

V. Conclusion

A pandemic brings about a moment of clarity: by heightening the risks at work in ordinary interactions with our neighbors, a virus makes the meaning and value of human life palpable. For Christians, that meaning and value can only be discerned with reference to the work and word of Jesus Christ. Our judgments about what might make human beings valuable would otherwise be governed by our own biases and preferences, which would invariably threaten the sanctity of the vulnerable. Affirming that humanity is made according to God's image and likeness provides a bulwark against such denigrating treatment: it underscores the infinite worth of every individual in their relatedness to God, and it calls us to walk in a manner that corresponds to the infinite love and honor God shows human beings in dying for them. Yet the ethical value of our infinite worth has rarely been specified, and invoking it in the midst of a pandemic creates its own moral hazards. My aim has been to disentangle the doctrine from both the claims that we must undertake a zero-risk stance toward imposing infections, and that we cannot make prudential, comparative judgments to save some people even if doing so means others might suffer or die. My hope is that specifying more precisely the role the doctrine plays in our theological anthropology and ethics will generate more precise policies in the midst of a pandemic, and so give more people time to fulfill their calling to bear witness to God's infinite love in their lives as only they can.

Endnotes

1. Feeding America, "The Impact of Coronavirus on Food Insecurity," FeedingAmerica.org, October 30, 2020, https://www.feedingamerica.org/research/coronavirus-hunger-research.

2. Centers for Disease Control and Prevention, "Preparing for COVID-19 in Nursing Homes," CDC.org, February 11, 2020, https://www.cdc.gov/coronavirus/2019-ncov/hcp/long-term-care.html.

3. "How Prisons in Each State Are Restricting Visits Due to Coronavirus," The Marshall Project, March 17, 2020, https://www.themarshallproject.org/2020/03/17/tracking-prisons-response-to-coronavirus.

4. For instances, see the discussion in Glenn K. Wakam et al., "Not Dying Alone—Modern Compassionate Care in the Covid-19 Pandemic," New England Journal of Medicine 382, no. 24 (2020): e88, https://doi.org/10.1056/NEJMp2007781. See also Katie Hafnner, "'A Heart-Wrenching Thing': Hospital Bans on Visits Devastates Families," The New York Times, March 29, 2020, https://www.nytimes.com/2020/03/29/health/coronavirus-hospital-visit-ban.html.

5. Stefanie DeLuca, Nick Papageorge, and Emma Kalish, "The Unequal Cost of Social Distancing," Johns Hopkins University of Medicine Coronavirus Resource Center, https://coronavirus.jhu.edu/from-our-experts/the-unequal-cost-of-social-distancing (accessed November 14, 2020).

6. Many of the arguments are distilled by Joel Zinberg, "Death by Policy: Mortality Statistics Show That Many People Have Died from Lockdown-oRelated Causes, Not from Covid-19," City Journal, July 9, 2020, https://www.city-journal.org/deadly-cost-of-lockdown-policies.

7. "Public health policies are entrenched with utilitarianism, the maximization of good for the highest number." Peter D. Murray and Jonathan R. Swanson, "Visitation Restrictions: Is It Right and How Do We Support Families in the NICU during COVID-19?" Journal of Perinatology 40, no. 10 (2020): 1576–81, https://doi.org/10.1038/s41372-020-00781-1. Rebecca Mitsos concurs: "Such policies are always developed for utilitarian reasons that sacrifice some benefits for individual patients and families to maximize benefits for the community. The community benefit accrues because such policies limit the spread of infection. During the COVID-19 pandemic, such policies also allow the conservation of scarce PPE. But they impose burdens on parents and may be psychologically detrimental for individual patients." Rebecca Mitsos, "Comments," in Alice K. Virani et al., "Benefits and Risks of Visitor Restrictions for Hospitalized Children During the COVID Pandemic," Pediatrics 146, no. 2 (2020): 4, https://doi.

org/10.1542/peds.2020-000786.

8. Mitsos, "Comments," 4. For a sophisticated account of what a utilitarian response might—and might not—require, see Julian Savulescu, Ingmar Persson, and Dominic Wilkinson, "Utilitarianism and the Pandemic," Bioethics 34, no. 6 (2020): 620–32, https://doi.org/10.1111/bioe.12771.

9. Albert Mohler, "Save Lives First, Repair the Economy Second: A Matter of Christian Priorities," AlbertMohler.com, March 27, 2020, https://albertmohler.com/2020/03/27/save-lives-first-repair-the-economy-second-a-matter-of-christian-priorities; Russell Moore, "God Doesn't Want Us to Sacrifice the Old," The New York Times, March 26, 2020, https://www.nytimes.com/2020/03/26/opinion/coronavirus-elderly-vulnerable-religion.html.

10. While utilitarians care only about well-being, they also can recognize that respecting liberty and rights can be important for overall well-being. Savulescu, Persson, and Wilkinson, "Utilitarianism and the Pandemic." Still, I take it that a Christian ethicist ought not be a utilitarian for many of the standard reasons held against the view.

11. John F. Kilner, Dignity and Destiny: Humanity in the Image of God (Grand Rapids, MI: Eerdmans, 2015), 315.

12. Andrew Bailey and Joshua Rasmussen point this problem out and argue that there are various types of "final value" that might accrue to a person. As such, comparative judgments between persons might be made on grounds other than their final value as a person. My own response to this problem will take a different tack. See Andrew M. Bailey and Joshua Rasmussen, "How Valuable Could a Person Be?" Philosophy and Phenomenological Research, July 15, 2020, https://doi.org/10.1111/phpr.12714.

13. As will become clear, much of what follows is influenced by Karl Barth. While there is much in Barth's theology and ethics with which I disagree, he has proved a valuable interlocutor. I have unpacked much of Barth's account in my as-of-yet unpublished dissertation. See Matthew Lee Anderson, "In Defence of Children: Pro- and Anti-Natalist Arguments in Moral Philosophy and Karl Barth" (PhD Thesis, University of Oxford, 2018). John Kilner also begins with the New Testament and with Christ in his weighty exploration of the doctrine, to which I am also much indebted. See Kilner, Dignity and Destiny, 52–82.

14. Karl Barth, Church Dogmatics 3.2 (Edinburgh: T & T Clark, 1960), 56.

15. Barth, Church Dogmatics 3.2, 56. Barth prioritizes the fact that humanity is for God. The distinctiveness of the creature "consists in the fact that it is for God" (70). At the same time, humanity "derives from the One who unceasingly comes to the very depths of his being in this way." (142) "Where do we come from? From the being, speaking and action of the eternal God

who has preceded us." (577) As I argue in my dissertation, Barth's emphasis on humanity's position as from God leaves the fact that we are also from humanity underdeveloped.

16. Barth, Church Dogmatics 3.2. See §47, and especially §47.4 and §47.5.

17. Barth, Church Dogmatics 3.2, §46.

18. Marc Cortez's exploration of these themes in Barth's thought is excellent. See Marc Cortez, Embodied Souls, Ensouled Bodies: An Exercise in Christological Anthropology and Its Significance for the Mind/Body Debate, (London: T&T Clark, 2011).

19. Karl Barth, Church Dogmatics 3.4, (Edinburgh: T & T Clark, 1960), 416.

20. Kilner, Dignity and Destiny, 89.

21. Kilner, Dignity and Destiny, 79 (emphasis original).

22. Cf. Kilner, Dignity and Destiny, 314. "One grasps the religious outlook upon the sanctity of human life only if he sees that this life is asserted to be surrounded by sanctity that need not be in a man; that the most dignity a man ever possesses is a dignity that is alien to him. . . . A man's dignity is an overflow from God's dealings with him, and not primarily an anticipation of anything he will ever be by himself alone." Paul Ramsey, "The Morality of Abortion," in Life or Death: Ethics and Options, ed. Edward Schils (Portland, OR: Reed College, 1968), 71. "That a man was and is and will be from and in the hand of God, this precisely, no less and no more, is his honour, the special honour of every man, which he cannot alter, which he cannot dimmish nor augment, which he cannot discard nor lose, which cannot be taken from him by others, just as he himself cannot create it or maintain it for himself." Barth correlates this 'honour' with human dignity. Barth, Church Dogmatics 3.4, 652–53.

23. "The individuality or singularity of each man is in the last analysis a reflection of the uniqueness of the offer [God makes] to him." And: "What is offered with such exclusiveness by God is surely worthy of honour, attention and reflection, even though its significance may not be immediately apparent." Barth, Church Dogmatics 3.4, 570, 572.

24. For a compelling argument that the resurrection of Jesus Christ is necessary to avoid this outcome, see Oliver O'Donovan, "Keeping Body and Soul Together," in Covenants of Life: Contemporary Medical Ethics in Light of the Thought of Paul Ramsey, ed. Kenneth L Vaux and Mark Stenberg (London: Springer, 2011), 35–56.

25. Such a "task" is possible even by those whose lives are spent in seriously disabling conditions, insofar as they teach others through their very presence the sometimes extraordinary demands love places upon us.

26. Note that neither irreplaceability nor uniqueness are the grounds for

our value. The infinite value of humanity by virtue of our relatedness to God is, instead, disclosed through that relatedness. For discussion on the differences, see Helen Watt, "The Dignity of Human Life: Sketching Out an 'Equal Worth' Approach," Ethics and Medicine 36, no. 1 (2020): 7–17. See also Stephen L. Brock, "Is Uniqueness at the Root of Personal Dignity? John Crosby and Thomas Aquinas," The Thomist: A Speculative Quarterly Review 69, no. 2 (2005): 173–201, https://doi.org/10.1353/tho.2005.0000; John F. Crosby, "The Twofold Source of the Dignity of Persons," Faith and Philosophy 18, no. 3 (2001): 292–306, https://doi.org/10.5840/faithphil200118326.

27. Barth, Church Dogmatics 3.2, §47.5.

28. It is certainly the case that death remains an intrinsic evil for the creature, as the sundering of body and soul are not conducive to its well-being. Yet this metaphysical account does not account for the way even "evils" (such as the harms inflicted by punishment) within the economy of salvation can be transformed into goods through their appropriate application. For a defense of the intrinsic badness of death within the Christian tradition, see David Albert Jones, Approaching the End: A Theological Exploration of Death and Dying, (Oxford: Oxford University Press, 2007).

29. Barth, Church Dogmatics 3.2, 632.

30. It is important to specify that family members are often an essential part of the team providing care to a patient, as they offer support and help deliberate about treatment options. See Joanna L. Hart et al., "Family-Centered Care During the COVID-19 Era," Journal of Pain and Symptom Management 60, no. 2 (2020): e93–97, https://doi.org/10.1016/j.jpainsymman.2020.04.017.

31. Fifteen hospitals allowed visitors at the end of life only. Thomas S. Valley et al., "Changes to Visitation Policies and Communication Practices in Michigan ICUs during the COVID-19 Pandemic," American Journal of Respiratory and Critical Care Medicine 202, no. 6 (2020): 883–85, https://doi.org/10.1164/rccm.202005-1706LE.

32. See Olga Khazan, "The Most American Failure Yet," The Atlantic, August 31, 2020, https://www.theatlantic.com/politics/archive/2020/08/contact-tracing-hr-6666-working-us/615637/.

33. Virani et al., "Benefits and Risks of Visitor Restrictions for Hospitalized Children During the COVID Pandemic," 4.

34. Teck Chuan Voo, Mathavi Senguttuvan, and Clarence C. Tam, "Family Presence for Patients and Separated Relatives During COVID-19: Physical, Virtual, and Surrogate," Journal of Bioethical Inquiry, August 25, 2020, https://doi.org/10.1007/s11673-020-10009-8.

35. The weaker moral claim such an outlook might generate is that someone

must be present at the moment of death; the stronger claim is that a family member must be present. The stronger claim is harder to demonstrate, insofar as it depends upon a differentiated account of the significance of hospice workers or chaplains to the individual's life and family members. I take it that family members are irreplaceable to dying in a way that other people are not, and as such, their presence bears unique witness to the irrepeatable significance of that life in a way that the presence of others cannot. The same might be said about friends or other partial moral bonds that are not role-specific the way hospice workers are. My thanks to an editor for flagging this issue.

36. Angela Coulter and Tessa Richards, "Care during Covid-19 Must Be Humane and Person Centred," BMJ, September 8, 2020, m3483, https://doi.org/10.1136/bmj.m3483.

37. "Denying visits or care by a family member may result in adverse and potentially long-term psychological effects for medically isolated patients, their families, and healthcare workers involved in their care." Voo, Senguttuvan, and Tam, "Family Presence for Patients and Separated Relatives During COVID-19," 2.

38. Questions of justice would inevitably arise, as families without financial or economic means to be so quarantined would be disadvantaged (though not more so than when end-of-life visits are prohibited outright).

39. For an overview of the doctrine, see Alison McIntyre, "Doctrine of Double Effect," in Stanford Encyclopedia of Philosophy, ed. Edward N. Zalta (December 24, 2018), https://plato.stanford.edu/archives/spr2019/entries/double-effect/.

40. While Kilner rejects what he calls "autonomy-based ethics" and "utilitarian ethics," the latter of which focuses on actions that are "beneficial to humanity," he suggests that there is a "role for such considerations, but it is secondary." Kilner, Dignity and Destiny, 103.

41. Jeff McMahan argues that the "default" "determines the nature of one's agency . . . [and] the nature of the agency affects the morality of the action." Jeff McMahan, "Causing People to Exist and Saving People's Lives," Journal of Ethics 17, no. 1–2 (2013): 16, https://doi.org/10.1007/s10892-012-9139-1.

42. Such a heuristic can only be that: a heuristic, and not an authoritative answer about the success of a policy. One reason we should ask no more of our criteria for public health considerations than partial insights is that the underlying causal explanations for any death are complicated, and a pandemic does not make them easier.

43. "An Incalculable Loss," The New York Times, May 27, 2020, https://www.nytimes.com/interactive/2020/05/24/us/us-coronavirus-deaths-100000.

html.

44. A social policy aimed at preventing deaths might be specified in a pandemic to preventing deaths by Covid-19, such that its success would be determined on that basis. In that case, the reference class or baseline for success would not be the raw number of deaths that happen over a given period, but the number of deaths that are attributable to this particular disease. There may be sound political or prudential reasons to adopt such a standard: a pathogen like SARS-CoV-2 is communicable in a way that deaths from suicide, a rise in poverty, or other sources are not. In that way, deaths by Covid-19 are a heuristic for how much a society contained the spread of the disease. Alternatively, one could adopt a standard that evaluates a response on the basis of "all cause" mortality, such that if deaths indirectly attributable to lockdowns, economic destruction, etc. exceed those lives saved, then the policy would be a failure. My point here is not to say that a doctrine of the image of God requires one judgment or the other—only that it might permit both.

45. The relevance of age to bioethics is often overlooked. I have discussed its importance as a background condition in making decisions about whether to treat or not treat elsewhere. It may be the case that in cases of limited health resources one might take age into account as a proxy for the burdens of treatment a person is likely to experience. However, this is distinct from discounting the badness of death on the basis of age. See Matthew Lee Anderson, "Indexing Burdens and Benefits of Treatment to Age: Revisiting Paul Ramsey's 'Medical Indications' Policy," Christian Bioethics (accepted for publication).

46. This is a variation of an argument I have made elsewhere. See my "Anti-abortionist Action Theory and the Asymmetry between Spontaneous and Induced Abortions," under review.

47. In Ethics at the Edges of Life, Paul Ramsey argues that under conditions of scarcity it might be permissible to set policies to treat or not treat various classes of patients. "A medical indications policy," he writes, "could go so far as to stipulate arbitrary lines to be drawn—for example, that no neonate below a designated weight and gestational age should be saved." However that line is drawn, physicians "could still be free within limits to the one side or the other to try to save or not to try to save the infant life." This policy still constitutes equal treatment of individuals, as it is a categorical determination of a class of patients. See Paul Ramsey, Ethics at the Edges of Life: Medical and Legal Intersections (New Haven, CT: Yale University Press, 1980), 264.

A PANDEMIC REMINDS US THAT WE ALL MATTER: BIOETHICS IN THE TIME OF COVID-19

CATHERINE GLENN FOSTER, MA, JD

I. Introduction

COVID-19 has presented innumerable vexing challenges for patients, caretakers, and lawmakers, not least in the realm of bioethics. Though pandemics have dotted the course of human history, COVID-19 is the most severe in recent memory and has led to a truly unprecedented disruption of our daily lives. As the public and lawmakers continue to grapple with how to live and operate in a world with COVID-19, we must be vigilant in ensuring that we proceed under an ethical framework that respects the equal worth and dignity of every human life. It is absolutely vital that the laws of our nation be derived from and guided by fundamental ethical principles—chiefly, a profound respect for human life as a gift of such inestimable worth that the loss of a single person diminishes every one of us.

We all matter. No matter the circumstances, where we come from, our location, our age, our dependence on those around us, or any other characteristics we may have, none of that changes or diminishes the one thing we all share—we maintain our fundamental right to life regardless of what we do. Nonetheless, the human right to life requires vigilant protection and defense against assault, against those ideologies that would seek to restrict it or tear it down. And so it is critical that we continue to strive towards true respect for this first and most important right.

There are four broad areas that present particular concerns for the realm of bioethics during COVID-19: 1) allocating scarce resources and prioritizing patient care, 2) caring for vulnerable populations and end-of-life dignity, 3) providing routine medical care, such as childbirth support and surgery, during a pandemic, and 4) countering abortion industry pressures during a pandemic. Examining each of these allows us to analyze and perhaps reevaluate the ethical bases of our healthcare system.

II. Allocating Scarce Resources and Prioritizing Patient Care

One of the initial concerns surrounding COVID-19 was the availability of ventilators and other intensive care unit (ICU) machinery. Though throughout the crisis thus far most hospitals in the U.S. have been able to meet the demand for ventilators, people were rightly concerned about how hospitals might make decisions about which patients would receive care from a ventilator, and which would not, when resources ran low. Pragmatically, the issue is also important because many jurisdictions are using ICU availability as one of the metrics to determine whether cities should maintain, loosen, or increase public restrictions—the more capacity in ICUs, the more likely a city is to be able to open.[1]

In March 2020, as the situation in Italy was worsening, I wrote in my capacity as President & CEO of Americans United for Life (AUL) in *The Federalist* urging President Trump to ensure that as many ventilators as possible would be available for the American people—arguing for the President to use "his executive power to mandate the rapid production of ventilators by major corporations," and that those companies "should redirect their production capacities to respond directly to the current crisis."[2] This strategy was, and remains, an important tool because there is a real risk that should COVID-19 cases skyrocket, or a future viral respiratory malady emerge, the U.S. will not have enough ventilators to care for all patients that need one.

A wide range of groups have expressed concerns about how hospitals might ration care, including those representing people with physical and/or mental disabilities, elder adults, and those who have a high BMI or other underlying health issues. Their concerns extend beyond how many ventilators are available. As more individuals requiring a lot of care end up in the hospital, people may be concerned about staffing shortages. Additionally, we have recently seen the first case of a COVID-19 patient getting a lifesaving double-lung transplant—leading to questions about which patients are most deserving of organ donations as time goes on.[3] And once a vaccine becomes available, the question of how to prioritize distribution will be up for debate. In all areas, each of the above-mentioned groups have reason for concern that if they end up in the hospital due to COVID-19, that they may be overlooked for care in favor of a younger or healthier patient.[4]

As we at AUL have written in our "Call for Unity on Ethical, Medical, and Political Principles in a Time of Crisis," creating a just distribution of scarce medical resources must focus on the welfare of the patient and how well a particular patient will respond to treatment. "Quality adjusted life years" are not an objective medical standard; they are inherently subjective and are bound to result in discriminatory effects like ageism, ableism, and racism. This system of rationing care has no place in the United States.[5]

Writing on "Ethical First Principles in a National Crisis," we have emphasized that "the cardinal virtues of charity and benevolence compel us to redouble our commitment to respecting all lives when many among us are vulnerable by virtue of their tender age, and others are made vulnerable by advancing age or infirmity." This requires an acceptance of the principle that "an enlightened society does not call the helpless, sick and infirm 'undignified' by virtue of their condition," and an understanding that "a government that implements a medical-legal regime that denies the value of any life based on its intrinsic vulnerability risks abolishing human dignity and human worth."[6]

What we must eschew is a utilitarian mindset that looks at which individuals have the most "life years" left and prioritizes their care over the care of others. In an extreme example, picture a 60-year-old and a 40-year-old who both need a ventilator, but only one is available. In a completely utilitarian approach, the 40-year-old would likely receive the ventilator because he would "benefit" the most from it; from a utilitarian perspective, because the statistical likelihood is that he could go on to live for more years than the 60-year-old, he is more "deserving" of the ventilator. This is the model we must avoid at all costs.

Instead of looking to who will live the longest, or who was healthier before contracting SARS-CoV-2, we should look to which patient is most likely to survive COVID-19 and be most likely to benefit from the particular treatment or therapy being considered. Charles LiMandri writes: "Federal law requires that decisions regarding the critical care of patients during the current crisis not discriminate on the basis of disability or age. In this respect, anticipated longevity or quality of life are inappropriate issues for consideration. Decisions must be made solely on clinical factors as to which patients have the greatest need and the best prospect of a good medical outcome. Therefore, disability and age should not be used as categorical exclusions in making these critical decisions."[7]

In other words, we should not be looking down the road 10 or 15 years, and not looking to how "valuable" a patient's life would be considered if they survive treatment. As Daniel Sulmasy writes, "A crisis can sometimes provoke cruelly cold rationality, thinking merely about maximizing the total 'quality-adjusted life years' saved. We must remember that all patients are of equal dignity and equally worthy of our efforts to help them."[8]

While it may seem far-fetched to be concerned that hospitals would adopt such a "cruelly cold" policy, renowned ethicists such as Peter Singer have recently endorsed this very proposition. He writes that using the World Health Organization's "disability-adjusted life year" to measure years lost by early death is a reasonable way to calculate losses. Singer states that anyone who would object to such a system based on the number of life-years lost is "perverse"—and, somewhat shockingly, that "we should not be misled by talk of 'saving lives.'"[9] This type of mentality swiftly morphs into discriminatory, ageist policies that don't value the inherent worth and dignity of elderly patients. Elder adults matter.

Thankfully, some states have already recognized how unethical treatment based on quality-adjusted life years is. In May 2020, Oklahoma banned rationing healthcare based on quality of life. Oklahoma's law notes that neither physical nor mental disabilities, age nor chronic illness diminishes a person's right to life, human dignity, or equal access to medical care.[10] Other states should take similar affirmative steps to codify anti-discrimination measures.

An ethos that proclaims some lives are worth more than others, and that some lives are fundamentally more worth living than others, is a toxic mentality that we must avoid at all costs. We must urge medical professionals to proactively develop ethical criteria for how to allocate care in case hospitals become overrun. And it is critical that those making decisions remember that all humans have equal worth and dignity and are all deserving of high-quality care. From there, we can debate the best means by which to allocate care when resources are scarce.[11]

III. Caring for Vulnerable Populations and End-of-Life Dignity

Elder adults and those with disabilities need and deserve special care, particularly during a pandemic. That care includes not only medical treatment, but humane, holistic care, to include reasonable procedures for visits and other contact with loved ones.

Improving Conditions for Elder Adults

COVID-19 has shown us the devastating effects of a pandemic on people in long-term care facilities. In most states, nursing home residents account for a dramatically disproportionate numbers of deaths. The AARP reported that as of June 1, 2020, over 38,000 nursing home residents and staff had died of COVID-19, roughly one-third of all deaths in the U.S. They also warned that this figure may actually be low because not all states are publicly reporting data on COVID-19 deaths.[12] By July 7, the *New York Times* reported that over 55,000 deaths—42% of all U.S. COVID-19 deaths—took place in nursing homes or long-term care facilities.[13]

The Centers for Medicare and Medicaid Services data shows that some states have particularly high levels of COVID-19 cases per resident.[14] In New Jersey, 46% of all nursing home residents have tested positive for COVID-19. In Connecticut and Massachusetts, it's around 37% of residents. Deaths per nursing home resident present similar concerns. In New Jersey, nearly 180 out of every 1,000 residents have died. In Connecticut and Massachusetts, the deaths total 115 out of every 1,000 residents. The impact of COVID-19 cannot be overstated.

Moreover, some states, like New York, have made devastating choices that have cost nursing home residents their lives. In March, New York decided to send 4,500 people infected with coronavirus to nursing homes, where they would finish recovering from the virus.[15] While this directive was eventually rolled back, the damage was done. While we do not yet know the full extent of nursing home deaths in New York, in January 2021 the New York attorney general announced that the administration had undercounted nursing home deaths due to COVID-19 by several thousand.[16]

The combination of older, frailer residents, coupled with close proximity to other residents and staff who cannot properly quarantine, has been the perfect storm to make nursing homes particularly deadly during this pandemic. Moving forward, states should reconsider policies that group people in nursing homes and be particularly wary of any suggestions to move recovering COVID-19 patients into nursing homes.

Another concerning element here is that within the already hard-hit nursing home population, nursing homes with predominantly minority residents seem to be hit even harder. As reported in the *New York Times*, nursing homes with predominately African-American or Latino residents "no matter their location, no matter their size, no matter their government rating—have been twice as likely to get hit by the coronavirus as those where the population is overwhelmingly white."[17] The *Times* article highlights that in Maryland, "80 percent of nursing homes with high black and Latino populations have been hit by the coronavirus, double the rate for homes with hardly any such residents."[18] It will be important for public health officials to examine the underlying causes of these disparities and address them accordingly.

However, even the tragedy of disproportionate deaths in nursing homes should not allow us to forget the human toll that living through COVID-19 will have on residents. We have already seen reflections about the devastation that isolation is taking on the elderly—unable to see their friends for communal meals, see their families on the week-ends, or attend church on Sundays, these nursing home residents and other elder adults who may already have less than ideal amounts of social interaction have essentially been in solitary confinement for months on end. The CDC has reported on the health risks of loneliness, noting that based on recent studies, we have reason to believe that it can lead to premature death, up to a 50% increased risk of dementia, a 29% increased risk of heart disease, and a 32% increased risk of stroke.[19] Moreover, we know that American adults may be more susceptible to these issues than their counterparts globally—Pew research shows that 27% of adults over 60 live alone in the U.S., compared to 16% of adults in other countries.[20]

Michael Toscano notes that "this is why extreme isolation is punishment—because it attacks our very nature. And this is why it cannot conceivably be considered a humane solution to the problems facing our elderly during the pandemic."[21] With no family and friends to check in on them, and nursing homes staffed more leanly, elderly residents are dying of neglect, starvation, and potentially despair. Those with dementia or other afflictions cannot process the change in their daily routines, and those who are of sound mind are devastated by the isolation they face. Even for the lucky ones who might be able to connect with family and friends on the phone or via FaceTime, electronic communication is no replacement for in-person interaction.[22]

The isolation resulting from full lockdown may even further increase the death rate, not only in nursing homes but also in the greater population.[23] The Well Being Trust & The Robert Graham Center put out a report estimating that the COVID-19 pandemic could lead to an additional 75,000 deaths due to alcohol and drug abuse. Benjamin Miller, Chief Strategy Officer for the Well Being Trust, says, "Undeniably, policymakers must place a large focus on mitigating the effects of COVID. However, if the country continues to ignore the collateral damage—specifically our nation's mental health—we will not come out of this stronger."[24] In a piece for *The Atlantic*, Olga Khazan writes about similar concerns; citing already increased suicides and overdoses among young adults, public health officials and mental health professionals are concerned about the additional deaths that isolation, job loss, and general instability may cause.[25]

Children are also vulnerable to the effects of prolonged isolation on their social and behavioral development. A Wall Street Journal article highlighted how throwing children off their routines and isolating them from their peers has a devastating impact. A mother, discussing her 11-year-old daughter, said that the COVID-19 lockdown "laid bare how important her personal relationships are to her daily happiness. . . . She is all about her friendships."[26] A pediatrician, Dimitri Christakis, noted that socially-distant playdates would not cut it—"social emotional learning happens when you are physically present with peers learning to negotiate and share. You can't do that over Zoom."[27] In the same article, professor of psychology Joseph P. Allen notes that "of all age groups, this virus is probably more socially devastating to teens than any other group. They are bored and they are lonely." He highlights that the teenage years require social interaction in order to "learn to manage issues of intimacy and loyalty and boundaries that are crucial to adult functioning."[28]

But in an institutional nursing home environment, these concerns about isolation and depression are coupled with issues of overworked staff as well as neglect and abuse. In one interview, Elise Amez-Droz spoke with Keziah Furth, who volunteered her services as a nurse at a nursing home in Boston as COVID-19 grew. Furth noted that staffing shortages were a huge issue:

> some nurses were out because they were sick themselves or had to be home to care for sick family members. Some were out

because of their own high-risk medical status. A large number of nursing assistants simply refused to come to work. . . . Most days I was the only nurse working with as many as 18 to 20 patients. It's a lot, and it's scary, and it's really hard to feel like you're doing the job well. [29]

Well-meaning nurses and staff like Furth have a difficult enough time under the new reality of COVID-19—more patients who need acute care, fewer staff to help with the job, and additional restrictive measures to prevent the spread of COVID-19.

On the other hand, other nursing homes and staff are coming under fire for neglecting and abusing residents. An ongoing investigation has revealed that New York City and New York State have not complied with a federal program in place to protect nursing home residents.[30] As reported in the *New York Post*, Queens has only six watchdogs to check in on 50,000 residents. These watchdogs—also known as ombudsmen—are tasked with identifying cases of abuse and neglect in nursing homes. But due to COVID-19, they have been prevented from checking in on these nursing homes and residents at all. An employee with the Milwaukee County Department on Aging noted that reports of abuse and financial exploitation are skyrocketing during COVID-19—saying the Department has seen a 15% increase in the first quarter of 2020.[31]

There are no easy solutions to finding a healthy way forward to reduce both nursing home deaths and the devastation of isolation, balancing individual well-being with the public good. Some have suggested finding a balance between quarantining residents to prevent the spread of COVID-19 with a more humane approach, where residents and families would have some level of choice in how much risk they are willing to accept in order to spend time together. Of course, if contact decisions are left up to each family connected to an institutional environment, it would be quite challenging to protect the whole nursing home. Charlie Camosy, Associate Professor of Bioethics at Fordham University, notes in a recent NPR interview: "I want to give someone the choice to be able to say it's more important for me to die here with my family and know I get to say goodbye to them then [sic] end up in a situation where I might be intubated, where I might be lost on a gurney in the hallway."[32] In order to support this, Camosy suggests another way: that we can increase support for home care and hospice, which will give families more options and more freedom to choose treatment options or palliative care based on the wishes of individuals, rather than by state mandate.[33]

Those with Disabilities Deserve Special Consideration

Much like nursing and assisted living homes, homes for developmentally and intellectually disabled individuals have been hit disproportionately hard by COVID-19. An Associated Press article notes that across the country, about 275,000 people with conditions like Down syndrome, cerebral palsy, and autism live in housing facilities.[34] Nearly 6,000 of them have already contracted COVID-19, and nearly 700 have died. And like much other reporting data, these numbers skew low because not all states, including large states like California and Texas, are reporting COVID-19 data. The Associated Press also notes that the underlying conditions at these facilities are already less than ideal: nearly 40% of Intermediate Care Facilities—which are the most common government-funded homes for the disabled—did not meet safety standards for preventing the spread of infections even before COVID-19 hit.

NPR reports that people with developmental or intellectual disabilities are dying at much higher rates than the general COVID-19-positive population—in New York, 16% of cases in disabled people led to death, compared to 6% of the state's cases overall, and in Pennsylvania that difference is 14% to 8%.[35] A study conducted by Scott Landes, Associate Professor of Sociology and Faculty Associate at the Aging Studies Institute at Syracuse University, has illuminated these disparities, showing that people with disabilities are more likely to have underlying health conditions that make them more susceptible to COVID-19, and that they are much more likely to live in group settings, frequently in close proximity to staff who enter their living space, which also contributes to the spread of COVID-19 because of the increased difficulties in social distancing.[36]

However, the news is not entirely bleak: Connecticut, at least, will finally allow patients with disabilities to have a support person accompany them to the hospital.[37] The Associated Press highlighted the story of Joan Parsons, a 73-year-old non-verbal woman who suffers from short-term memory loss yet was denied access to a support person. Her daughter said that no one in the family could see or communicate with her as she was in the hospital with COVID-19. Parsons' family alleged that she was treated poorly—physically and mentally—in the hospital: restrained, unable to consent to several tests, and doctors missed several issues when caring for her. In response to this case, Connecticut Governor Ned Lamont signed an executive order allowing disabled patients to have a caretaker with them in the hospital in hopes of achieving better patient advocacy. Roger Severino, Director of the HHS Office for Civil Rights, noted, "we've heard many heart-wrenching stories of people literally dying alone during the crisis. . . . This goes a big step toward assuring that people with disabilities are not left alone and not left to fend for themselves when reasonable accommodations can be made."[38]

Ethically Responding to Our Need to Visit and Make Accommodations for Loved Ones

Even in normal times, it can be difficult for families to visit with loved ones who are sick. During a pandemic, it's become nearly impossible for family to visit relatives before they pass away, grieve in person with friends, or even have a proper funeral.

In a poignant piece, journalist Christine Rousselle reflected on her father's sudden illness and subsequent passing.[39] Though he lived in Maine, where there had been very few cases of COVID-19 reported, once her father went into the hospital after a heart attack, no one was allowed to visit him. She and her family received pushback from the hospital when they requested her father receive Last Rites—Catholic sacraments that are traditionally bestowed to the dying. It wasn't until the day before Rousselle's father passed away that the hospital would allow a single visitor to see him—and it wasn't until the organ donation team lobbied for *two* visitors that both Rousselle and her aunt were able to say goodbye to her father. The funeral planning process was just as stressful—technically only allowed to have ten people at the outdoor gravesite, Rousselle was looking over her shoulder, hoping the police would not come and ticket them for having closer to 20 people in attendance. There were plenty of other, smaller, struggles along the way—scheduling a flight when airlines have cut many of their routes, not being able to buy a black dress for the unexpected funeral due to store closures, and having to wave through the window at friends who dropped off care packages and flowers rather than hugging and visiting with them.

Rousselle's story has perhaps been circulated so widely because so many families can connect with it and empathize. Even in the best of times, planning a funeral and grieving a lost family member can seem unbearable. Doing so during a pandemic, without the support of friends and family and without proper closure, borders on inhumane.

Members of the AUL team have had our own experiences with how quickly the otherwise normal grieving process turned into what might aptly be described as a "drive-by funeral." In early March, I attended a funeral in Rhode Island just before the physical-distancing recommendations for COVID-19 kicked in. Attendees were urged not to shake hands, but we were able to gather for the funeral and have lunch with the family afterwards. Mere weeks later, when attending a second funeral in Alabama, attendance was limited, we were directed to remain in our cars—many yards away—during the graveside service, and we were unable to hear the eulogy. It seemed like before we could even figure out that the burial service had started, it was already over; we drove away unable to mourn with family, let alone visit with them or share a meal.

As we move forward through COVID-19, we must reevaluate how we allow people to access their loved ones in the hospital and give them some semblance of a normal grieving period should they pass away. We can do this with a sober perspective about how big a risk COVID-19 is to the public. This will require ongoing studies on COVID-19 transmission indoors versus outdoors, mask efficacy, and other considerations, but it is clear that we should pursue options that allow people to bury loved ones with the support of family and friends rather than leaving them to bear that weight alone.

We must work to ensure better care for our elder adults and those with disabilities and take seriously the claims that isolation coupled with the stress of living through a pandemic will wreak havoc not only on nursing home and assisted living residents, but also on everyday adults and even children. We must work to find a safe middle ground—where we have as few residents in nursing homes as possible, prioritize and incentivize home care, and allow those residents to still be able to safely socialize with friends and family. Isolating anyone—particularly elder adults—for months on end with no means of human interaction is an inhumane response.

Protecting Vulnerable Populations from Pressure Towards Death

Another disheartening result of COVID-19 isolation is increased lobbying for euthanasia and physician-assisted suicide. Alex Schadenberg, Executive Director of the Euthanasia Prevention Coalition, has warned about growing demands by the euthanasia lobby to expand access to killing by physician in Canada and Massachusetts. Indeed, in May—in the midst of the COVID-19 crisis—a suicide bill in Massachusetts moved forward, making it out of committee in an 11-to-6 vote. The president of a pro-euthanasia group, Compassion and Choices, specifically invoked COVID-19 as a reason to pass the bill, saying "COVID-19 has shined a spotlight on the importance of a compassionate death, and we thank the public health committee for prioritizing this legislation . . . . We urge legislative leaders to hold floor votes on the bill ASAP so that more Massachusetts residents will have the option of a peaceful end should their suffering become intolerable."[40] And we know that if states expand access to suicide by physician, many elderly, disabled, or otherwise vulnerable COVID-19 patients will be pressured into choosing it.

After all, euthanasia without consent is already happening in Europe. Attorney Wesley Smith, Chair and Senior Fellow at the Discovery Institute's Center on Human Exceptionalism, describes the particularly chilling story of a Dutch woman who was killed even after she affirmatively declared she did not want to die.[41] The doctor, who euthanized the woman by slipping sedatives into her coffee before administering the drugs, recently stated, "If you asked her 'what would you think if I were to help you to die?', she looked bewildered and said: 'That is going a bit far!' I saw in her eyes that she didn't understand it anymore."[42] This doctor admitted to killing her patient after that patient declared she did not want to die, yet was cleared of murder charges. Smith puts the implications well: "This involuntary euthanasia was motivated by bigotry against people with dementia, masked as compassion. What other conclusion can we reach? That she was no longer *compos mentis*, so her opinion about her own life was unimportant?"[43] And being that this case took place before COVID-19—long before concerns about too few resources and scarce patient care—how many more people will be killed because fighting COVID-19, or the long recovery process after it, isn't deemed "worth it" by medical professionals?

Perhaps even more concerning, activists are now pushing for telemedicine euthanasia via Zoom. Smith noted that new guidelines published by The American Clinicians Academy on Medical Aid in Dying included formal guidelines that would allow doctors to prescribe euthanasia drugs via Skype, Zoom, and similar technologies. Smith puts it well: "This means that assisted suicides will be facilitated by doctors who never actually treated patients for their underlying illness, who may be ignorant of their family situations and personal histories, and who have never met their patients in the flesh." [44]

IV. Providing Routine Medical Care During a Pandemic: Childbirth and Surgery

COVID-19 has certainly presented unique challenges as we work together, but physically distanced, to live through the pandemic, and to appropriately honor and mourn those who have died. But COVID-19 is also impacting our ability to access routine medical care, such as pregnancy and childbirth care, and non-emergency surgeries.

COVID-19 has upended the process of being pregnant and giving birth—from making it impossible for partners to attend prenatal visits to real concerns that women would have to give birth alone, without a birth partner in the room. And we do not yet fully understand the impact of COVID-19 during pregnancy—is it dangerous for pregnant women, or children in the womb? Will a vaccine be safe for pregnant women or children to receive once it is developed?

Dr. Leana Wen, an emergency physician, shared some advice and facts with the website What to Expect.[45] Dr. Wen suggested that flexibility will be key for expecting mothers—for example, she suggests talking to doctors about which appointments should be handled in person and which could be switched to telemedicine appointments so that the potential for exposure to COVID-19 can be reduced. She also noted that there is a lot we simply still do not know about the virus—for example, we are not sure whether pregnant women are more susceptible to contract COVID-19, and we are not sure whether preborn children are at risk if a mother does contract it. The data is simply too limited to tell. Thankfully, researchers at the University of Utah are conducting a nationwide study to look at the effects of COVID-19 on pregnant women and women who have recently given birth.[46] Part of that research will involve tracking over 1,500 pregnant women who have been confirmed positive for COVID-19. This research should allow pregnant women to have better information about the risks associated with COVID-19 and pregnancy.

Thankfully, the most extreme measures, such as forcing women to give birth alone, seem to either not have been implemented outside of the hardest-hit areas or rolled back after much public outcry. But even though many hospitals have policies in place allowing a single birth partner to be present during delivery, some hospitals will not allow those individuals to be present during caesarian sections because it requires using an additional set of PPE and surgical gear. There are also concerns that women may be forced out of hospitals more quickly than they should be after giving birth to lessen their exposure to COVID-19. Alternatively, more women are choosing home births, even in higher-risk situations, in lieu of going to a hospital.[47]

While home births are typically perfectly safe for mothers and their children, we have already seen some examples of a home birth sparked by coronavirus concerns leading to tragic results. In an interview with Good Morning America, Kara Keough Bosworth recounts how her son passed away after a rare complication during childbirth. She said, "As I found out that the doula wasn't going to be able to be there, I started to get really anxious. In some cities, people weren't even allowed to have their birth partner in the delivery room with them. And then I started to get really anxious and really afraid."[48] Bosworth changed her birth plan, planning to labor at home for as long as possible before going to the hospital for a delivery, after what her own OB considered an "uneventful and boring pregnancy." She recounts thinking, "What if I spiked a fever because that's sometimes a normal part of giving birth, and then I get my baby taken from me? And I mean the irony now looking back is, I don't have my baby now. But the fear of all of that compounded so much." During birth, her son suffered from shoulder dystocia—a rare complication where his head was birthed, but his shoulder was stuck inside of Bosworth's pelvis. Miraculously, her son lived for a few days despite not having had a heartbeat for over 45 minutes, but eventually he passed away from complications of the dystocia. We do not definitively know whether things would have gone differently for Bosworth and her son had she moved forward with her original in-hospital birth plan. But it is clear that the stress and complications that come from having to make last-minute decisions about previously well-laid birth plans can lead to devastating results.

Sadly, the youngest among us are not spared from this tragedy either. While the ethical concerns surrounding surrogacy, and perhaps particularly international surrogacy, inherently merit concern and debate, COVID-19 has made the surrogacy process even more dangerous. COVID-19-related travel restrictions have resulted in parents who paid surrogates in Ukraine to carry and birth babies not being able to see those children for months, with the children often left to institutional care as they await their intended parents.

One clinic in Ukraine drew international attention when it ended up with over 100 babies in a nursery, stuck there, with no way for their biological parents to reach them. The babies had been born as the Ukraine was in lockdown from COVID-19—meaning the biological parents have not been able to enter the country and bring their children home. A *Guardian* essay highlights the horror of the situation: "anxious parents check on the children they have not yet met via video calls, and others have sent audio recordings of their voices to soothe the children." [49] Only recently have some of the parents been given access to the country—a *TIME* article suggests about 31 parents have been able to bring their children home.[50] But given what we know about the earliest needs of childhood development, this situation could be disastrous.[51] Infants need socialization and bonding from their first day on Earth. Having dozens of children in a hospital-like setup for weeks or months, without their parents or a one-on-one caretaker, could lead to bonding and developmental issues down the road.

In dealing with COVID-19 and tackling the issue of personal protective equipment (PPE) shortages, states have had to decide what counts as a necessary versus an elective procedure and what could or should be postponed. In the end, critical screenings such as colonoscopies and mammograms were frequently deemed "elective," and even more acute medical issues like dental surgery, hip replacements, and other treatments have not been considered necessary procedures. A *New Yorker* article written by Dr. Alessandra Colaianni recounts the chaos of these suddenly cancelled surgeries, with hospital staff unsure of whether surgeries were scheduled or not and patients not getting the message that their operations were put on hold. She asks, "Should we perform an urgent cancer operation on a patient with underlying pulmonary disease, when there is a possibility that the patient may need an I.C.U. bed after surgery? Is it ethical to delay that case, when the tumor may grow and strangle the patient, potentially forcing an emergency airway intervention with no time for COVID-19 testing?"[52] While we do not know the full extent of the impact that these delays will have, we should watch closely to see whether we see a spike in delayed diagnoses or worse outcomes due to delayed treatment. We must also be vigilant and help doctors protect themselves and other medical personnel from contracting COVID-19.

Moreover, some have expressed concern that individuals with medical emergencies, such as potential heart attacks and strokes, are avoiding calling 911 or going to the emergency room for fear of contracting COVID-19 or because of a mistaken belief that hospitals do not have the capacity to treat non-COVID-19 patients. An ICU doctor, Alex Hakim, writing for *The Federalist*, warns, "There is so much fear of going to the ER right now that, without any exaggeration, I have seen multiple major illnesses leading to death that could have been easily prevented by patients coming in earlier. Family members told me the patient was reluctant to come and get exposed."[53]

Moving forward, governments and medical professionals must work together to ensure that enough PPE is available so that these necessary screenings can be accessible even in the midst of a COVID-19 spike. Additionally, they should be sure to communicate to the public which hospitals have the capacity to treat non-COVID-19 emergency issues so that people are not left waiting to seek treatment until it is too late.

V. Countering Abortion Industry Pressures During a Pandemic

When it comes to abortion, the abortion lobby has continued to push for government funding for abortions, for abortion to be classified as a necessary rather than an elective procedure during the pandemic, and for expanded availability of abortion. None of these efforts are in line with public opinion. William Saletan, writing for *Slate*, summarizes, "In every poll, a plurality of Americans opposes public funding of abortions. In every poll but one, that plurality is a majority. . . . These polls aren't close. The average gap between the pro-funding and anti-funding positions is 19 percentage points."[54]

And in a poll conducted in late May and early June—well after the start of COVID-19—a majority of Americans think abortion should either not be permitted at all, or only available in certain cases.[55] This response is similar to that of a poll taken at the same time last year; according to Michael New, the results represent "a one-point gain on this question compared with last year's CBS News poll."[56] And the poll saw a four-point drop in a question about whether the U.S. Supreme Court should keep the *Roe v. Wade* decision "as-is." Overall, the survey results suggest that the abortion lobby is wrong when it claims that Americans want expanded access to abortion due to the effects of COVID-19.

Unfortunately, there is cause for concern about the number of women seeking abortions. Florida, for example, has indicated that the number of abortions performed in the state is 3.5% higher now than it was at this time last year. And so in the same *National Review* article, Dr. Michael New argues that we should increase funding and support for pregnancy centers—many of which may have seen a drop-off in volunteers or resources given the shutdowns—and reminds us that "during this time of disruption, there remain plenty of ways for pro-lifers to build a culture of life."[57]

Planned Parenthood Gets a Payout from the Paycheck Protection Program

The Coronavirus Aid, Relief, and Economic Security (CARES) Act, passed in March 2020 in response to the COVID-19 pandemic, created the Paycheck Protection Program to distribute money to small businesses struggling to keep their payrolls afloat during lockdown. The parameters of this program do not allow affiliates of organizations with over 500 employees to receive funding. These rules were clearly established when the bill was passed, and Planned Parenthood undeniably has well over 500 employees. Despite this clarity in the law and the stark difference between the behemoth of Planned Parenthood and the many millions of small businesses trying to stay afloat, *thirty-seven* Planned Parenthood affiliates applied for funding totaling $80 million in loans from the program. For example, Planned Parenthood of Southwest Central Florida received about $2 million in funding, and the Planned Parenthood affiliate in Washington DC received more than $1.3 million.[58]

After the Susan B. Anthony List became aware of these applications, it alerted the Small Business Administration to the problem. And nearly 100 Senators and Representatives voiced their concern over the Planned

Parenthood affiliate applications in an April 30, 2020 letter to the Small Business Administration.[59] They note that Planned Parenthood has over 16,000 employees nationwide and that Planned Parenthood "makes no attempt to hide its control over its affiliates nationwide." For instance, Planned Parenthood describes its affiliates as "local offices," and its by-law structure allows for Planned Parenthood to control these affiliates by handing down policies and practices that the affiliates must follow. These affiliates would be fully aware of their status, particularly because Planned Parenthood imposes a "Manual of Medical Standards and Guidelines" with which all of these affiliates are required to comply or risk having their affiliate status jeopardized. Most telling, the members of Congress highlighted that after the CARES Act passed the Senate, Planned Parenthood Action Fund released a statement criticizing the bill for giving the Small Business Administration "broad discretion to exclude Planned Parenthood affiliates . . . and deny them benefits under the new small business loan program."[60] There was no confusion or ambiguity about Planned Parenthood affiliates' non-eligibility for these loans.

Senator Josh Hawley of Missouri wrote his own letter to the Small Business Administration: "From the very beginning, Planned Parenthood's exclusion from the Paycheck Protection Program has been very well known and the subject of much discussion. . . . In light of the clear text of the CARES Act and Planned Parenthood's own admission that every one of its offices are affiliated with each other, it is hard to conclude anything other than that Planned Parenthood committed fraud."[61]

While this dispute is still unresolved, and there has not been a definitive decision on whether the applications were in fact fraudulent, it seems that the Small Business Administration has contacted the Planned Parenthood affiliates that inappropriately applied for funding to inform them that they could face significant penalties in addition to mandatory repayment of the loans.[62]

The Abortion Industry Sues for an Exception to Delaying Elective Surgeries

As mentioned above, in the midst of the COVID-19 crisis, many important medical procedures such as colonoscopies, mammograms, dental surgeries, and knee replacements have been deemed "elective" and put on hold. There are several reasons for these classifications and delays: to protect patients who may contract COVID-19 from a hospital stay or visit to a doctor's office, to keep resources such as PPE available for those in emergency rooms and COVID-19 wards in the critical early days of the pandemic, and to prevent the spread of COVID-19 from patients to doctors in non-emergency scenarios. Despite the need for these safeguards, the abortion industry will not budge, and continues to put women, doctors, and the public in harm's way by demanding that abortions be just as available, on demand, even during this public health crisis. U.S. Representative Ted Budd put it this way: "Abortion businesses that continue to operate are putting everyone at risk—women, employees, emergency responders who are left picking up the pieces when women suffer injuries and complications from abortions, and the general public."[63]

Litigation is ongoing, and the situation will remain fluid as COVID-19 restrictions ebb and flow. But as an example of how courts are handling these bans, we can look to a Fifth Circuit opinion from April. Governor Abbott of Texas, like many other governors, had restricted which medical procedures could take place while COVID-19 cases increased in his state. He did this to preserve hospital beds and supplies, and to ensure that PPE remained accessible to front-line professionals battling COVID-19. Weighing all the factors, Texas categorized non-emergency abortions as elective procedures. And while the trial-level District Court was willing to overturn Texas' categorization of abortion as a non-medically necessary procedure, the appellate court disagreed, determining that abortion should be treated just as other procedures were, and that the restrictions could stay in place.[64]

In Arkansas, the government required that women receive a negative COVID-19 test before being able to receive a surgical abortion.[65] While a federal District Court judge issued a temporary restraining order (TRO) on that requirement, the Eighth Circuit ruled that the health and safety concerns surrounding COVID-19 were great enough that the TRO should be lifted, and that the policy could stay in place.[66] The court noted that this was a facially-neutral directive, meaning that anyone seeking a surgical procedure would need a negative COVID-19 test, and reasoned that surgical abortions require the use of PPE, which has been in short supply for medical professionals on the front lines of the COVID-19 pandemic. It will be important to watch how other Circuit Courts rule on this issue because their guidance will be instructive to state governments who want to put similar safeguards in place.

Sadly, in a similarly dangerous situation in Missouri, Planned Parenthood recently obtained a court order that would allow its abortion business in St. Louis to continue operating even though it did not meet Missouri's health and safety standards. The state law requires an obstetric examination three days before any abortion in order to ensure that the procedure would be safe for the woman—for example, to confirm that the pregnancy is not ectopic. However, the clinic in Missouri failed to comply with that regulation and failed to document failed abortions—further putting women at risk. Despite these failings, the Missouri Department of Health and Senior Services decided to renew the facility's license.

This Grave Public Health Crisis Is Absolutely No Reason to Expand the Violence of Abortion

Both surgical and chemical abortions have been impacted by the coronavirus pandemic, as broadening access to at-home chemical abortions will only increase the already significant risks they pose to women. The chemical abortion pill is a regime of two drugs, mifepristone and misoprostol. In most states, a woman takes the first pill on-site and the second pill later at home. Though advocates tout the abortion pill as being risk-free and without complications to women, the facts do not support their claims. Instead, many reports show that the abortion pill is dangerous for women. Since it began tracking the data, the FDA has reported 22 deaths, nearly 800 hospitalizations, over 400 women experiencing so much blood loss they required transfusions, and over 300 infections related to the abortion pill.[67] In fact, the abortion pill has a higher rate of hemorrhage and sepsis than surgical abortion. A 2009 study showed that after chemical abortion, hemorrhage occurs 15.6% of the time; incomplete abortions, 6.7%; and surgery after a failed abortion, 5.9% of the time.[68]

Clearly, this combination of drugs is dangerous for women, particularly when being pushed at a time when the medical system is on the brink of being overwhelmed due to COVID-19. In a time when hospital resources are already strained, pushing women to use chemical abortion pills at home could lead to catastrophic results. If women who take the abortion pill have complications due to hemorrhaging, infection, or failure of the abortion pill—which would require removing retained products left inside the woman's body—they would have to be transported to a hospital, potentially be exposed to COVID-19, and put further strain on hospital resources.

Despite the clear risks involved with taking the abortion pill, pro-abortion activists are pushing to loosen chemical abortion regulations and allow for telemedicine abortions. Under their proposal, a woman would video chat with a doctor who would then either mail the abortion pills to her home or call them into a pharmacy, where someone could pick them up. This proposal does not allow for the necessary physical examination to determine gestational age and confirm that the pregnancy is not ectopic, and is not medically sound; it places already vulnerable women at even greater risk. Passing over these minimal safeguards is dangerous. Ultrasounds are the most effective way to accurately date pregnancies and to confirm that pregnancies are not ectopic. Additionally, in-person confirmation of pregnancy and identity are some of the only safeguards to ensure that women are not being coerced into undergoing a chemical abortion. And women need to visit clinics after chemical abortions to confirm that the abortion has been completed and assess any potential complications that may have developed from using the chemical abortion pill.

For example, Rh factor testing early in pregnancies can help prevent future infertility. Writing for the *Washington Examiner*, Kristi Stone Hamrick notes that "in its 2020 Clinical Policy Guidelines for abortion care, the National Abortion Federation's team of experts admits that the standard of care has been to determine a woman's Rh status and treat her accordingly. Yet their recommendation was that in pregnancies less than 56 days . . . chemical abortion sales associates may 'forego Rh testing.'"[69]

As AUL's Katie Glenn pointed out in a webinar in May 2020, the push for expanded chemical abortion via telemedicine is "a clear case of abortionists prioritizing the convenience and cost-saving of at-home abortion over the safety and lives of women."[70]

Despite all this, abortion activists continue to push for chemical abortion expansion. The company "TelAbortion," a commercial operator that operates in 13 states and contracts with for-profit abortion companies, reported that its business doubled in March and April; it is working to expand.[71] The ACLU has filed a lawsuit in Maryland, trying to roll back protections that keep women safe.[72] There are grave concerns over the illegal sale of abortion-inducing drugs sold over the internet, many of which are manufactured overseas and shipped into the U.S. without oversight by doctors; in a letter to the U.S. Food and Drug Administration, pro-life groups note that several websites are circumventing the regulatory safeguards that currently control how abortion pills are dispensed in the U.S.[73] Alexis McGill Johnson, President and CEO of the Planned Parenthood Federation of America, said that "it is actually a silver lining in this pandemic, that Planned Parenthood and many other health providers have actually been able to really lean into telehealth infrastructure and provide service."[74]

Not surprisingly, the Abortion Pill Rescue Network—which assists women who regret their decision to begin chemical abortions—reported that March 2020 was its busiest month ever.[75] The Abortion Pill Rescue Network helps women by connecting them with local medical providers who are able to prescribe ongoing dosages or progesterone in hopes of stopping the abortion.

But we in the United States are not alone in having to oppose chemical abortion expansion; in response to the COVID-19 pandemic, the UK has instituted a new pilot program called "Pills by Post." After consulting over the telephone—not in person—a woman is mailed pills that she then takes at home to induce a chemical abortion. She receives no in-person confirmation of her pregnancy, no ultrasounds, no confirmation that she's early along enough in the pregnancy to use the chemical abortion pill, no necessary follow-up treatment, and no confirmation of her identity. The program's own website notes, "you will NOT be contacted by BPAS to find out if your treatment has worked. You need to complete the 'self-assessment checklist' below to ensure your treatment has worked and that you are no longer pregnant."[76] In effect, this means that a woman would never have to see a follow-up healthcare provider to ensure that the abortion was successful and is left to fend for herself in determining whether she requires follow-up care. Women deserve better than this abdication of medical responsibility.

Unsurprisingly, the UK government has already uncovered cases of abuse just in the first few weeks of its telemedicine abortion program. For instance, the government is investigating the abortion of a 28-week baby by chemical abortion. That's four weeks beyond the UK's 24-week abortion limit, and 18 weeks past the limit for using the chemical abortion pill. This is just one of several cases where women have taken the drugs well after the 70-day cutoff.[77]

The facts are clear: telemedicine abortion enriches unscrupulous doctors while endangering the physical and emotional health of women and girls. While telemedicine has many beneficial applications, especially during the COVID-19 outbreak, abortion is not one of them.

VI. Conclusion

Keeping these ethical concerns in mind, where are we supposed to go from here? The response to COVID-19 is unlike anything we have seen in our lifetime. We are voluntarily shutting down much of the U.S. economy, worrying that ICUs across the country will be overrun with patients, and sifting through the very little information we have about how to prevent the spread of a virus that we do not fully understand—and potentially preparing to do it all again should additional waves overwhelm states before a vaccine is made widely available. In order to tackle COVID-19 ethically, all stakeholders, including federal and state governments, medical professionals, and patients and families, must be urged to approach the situation with a perspective framed around human dignity.

Taking measures to reduce COVID-19 cases without respecting the autonomy and equal worth and value of every human life is simply not an option we should pursue. As we begin to see additional policy and treatment proposals put on the table, we have to ask ourselves whether all patients, regardless of age and underlying health, are being treated equally. We have to assess whether we have better, more humane options than keeping elderly residents and other vulnerable individuals locked away in residential facilities with no outside contact. And we have to challenge the abortion lobby and protect the women they would seek to take advantage of by promoting unsafe practices like unregulated at-home abortions. Only when we take seriously the first principles of general welfare—most importantly, a deep respect for human life—will we be able to effectively combat COVID-19 and all of its ethical complications.

Most of all, we must remember the most fundamental truth of our shared existence. Even when in trying times, even when we are facing something new, and even when we are scared, we all matter.

Endnotes

1. See, e.g., Kristina Fiore et al., "Here's How States Actually Determine Reopening—See the Criteria Each Used to Get Their Economies Back on Track, and How That Differs from Federal Guidance," MedPage Today, June 5, 2020, https://www.medpagetoday.com/publichealthpolicy/healthpolicy/86916; J. Ryne Danielson, "Surging Virus, Falling ICU Capacity May Delay IL Reopening," Patch, April 20, 2021, https://patch.com/illinois/chicago/surging-virus-falling-icu-capacity-may-delay-il-reopening; Mike Roe, "CA COVID-19 Update: How ICU Projections Led to Reopening; 'If You Miss a Friend, You Can Go Out to Eat,'" LAist, Jan. 26, 2021, https://laist.com/news/public-health-mark-ghaly-covid-19-coronavirus-purple-tier; Massachusetts Department of Public Health, "Reopen Approach for Acute Care Hospitals," May 25, 2020, https://www.mass.gov/doc/dph-phase-1-reopening-guidance-acute-care-hospitals/download; Carri W. Chan & Hayley B. Gershengorn, "A Call to Revise CDC Guidelines for Reopening," The Hill, June 18, 2020, https://thehill.com/opinion/healthcare/503345-a-call-to-revise-cdc-guidelines-for-reopening.

2. Catherine Glenn Foster, "Trump Needs to Demand That Major Corporations Start Making Ventilators, Stat," The Federalist, March 27, 2020, https://thefederalist.com/2020/03/27/trump-needs-to-demand-that-major-corporations-start-making-ventilators-stat/.

3. Christine Herman, "1st-Known U.S. Lung Transplant for COVID-19 Patient Performed in Chicago," NPR, June 12, 2020, https://www.npr.org/sections/health-shots/2020/06/12/875486356/first-known-u-s-lung-transplant-for-covid-19-patient-performed-in-chicago.

4. Mike Baker and Sheri Fink, "At the Top of the Covid-19 Curve, How do Hospitals Decide Who Gets Treatment?" New York Times, March 31, 2020, https://www.nytimes.com/2020/03/31/us/coronavirus-covid-triage-rationing-ventilators.html.

5. "Americans United for Life Calls for Unity on Ethical, Medical, and Political Principles in a Time of Crisis," Americans United for Life, April 15, 2020 https://aul.org/2020/04/15/americans-united-for-life-calls-for-unity-on-ethical-medical-and-political-principles-in-a-time-of-crisis/.

6. "Ethical First Principles in a National Crisis," Americans United for Life, April 10, 2020, https://aul.org/2020/04/10/ethical-first-principles-in-a-national-crisis/.

7. Quoted in Alexandra DeSanctis, "Age Discrimination and Rationing during the Coronavirus Crisis," National Review, March 25, 2020, https://www.nationalreview.com/corner/age-discrimination-and-rationing-during-the-coronavirus-crisis/?itm_source=parsely-api.

8. Daniel Sulmasy, "Respirators, Our Rights, Right and Wrong: Medial Ethics

in an Age of Coronavirus, New York Daily News, March 22, 2020, https://www.nydailynews.com/opinion/ny-oped-respirators-right-and-wrong-20200322-niu3aosa7ffzjfg7led3lymb7a-story.html.

9. Peter Singer, "Is Age Discrimination Acceptable?" Project Syndicate, June 10, 2020, https://www.project-syndicate.org/commentary/when-is-age-discrimination-acceptable-by-peter-singer-2020-06.

10. Wesley J. Smith, "Oklahoma Bans 'Quality of Life' Health-Care Rationing," National Review, May 26, 2020, https://www.nationalreview.com/corner/oklahoma-bans-quality-of-life-health-care-rationing/.

11. Robert C. Koons, "Can We Measure the Value of Human Lives in Dollars? Somber Calculations in a Time of Plague," Public Discourse, March 31, 2020, https://www.thepublicdiscourse.com/2020/03/61900/.

12. Emily Paulin, "How to Track COVID-19 Nursing Home Cases and Deaths in Your State," AARP, June 1, 2020, https://www.aarp.org/caregiving/health/info-2020/coronavirus-nursing-home-cases-deaths.html.

13. "More than 40% of U.S. Coronavirus Deaths are Linked to Nursing Homes," New York Times, July 7, 2020, https://www.nytimes.com/interactive/2020/us/coronavirus-nursing-homes.html.

14. "COVID-19 Nursing Home Data," CMS.gov, June 21, 2020, https://data.cms.gov/stories/s/COVID-19-Nursing-Home-Data/bkwz-xpvg/.

15. Bernard Condon, Jennifer Peltz, and Jim Mustian, "AP Count: Over 4,500 Virus Patients Sent to NY Nursing Homes," Associated Press, May 22, 2020, https://abcnews.go.com/Health/wireStory/ap-count-4300-virus-patients-ny-nursing-homes-70825470.

16. Jesse McKinley and Luis Ferré-Sadurní, "N.Y. Severely Undercounted Virus Deaths in Nursing Homes, Report Says," The New York Times, Jan. 28, 2021, https://www.nytimes.com/2021/01/28/nyregion/nursing-home-deaths-cuomo.html.

17. Robert Gebeloff et al., "The Striking Racial Divide in How Covid-19 Has Hit Nursing Homes," The New York Times, May 21, 2020, https://www.nytimes.com/article/coronavirus-nursing-homes-racial-disparity.html.

18. Gebeloff et al., "The Striking Racial Divide in How Covid-19 Has Hit Nursing Homes."

19. CDC, "Loneliness and Social Isolation Linked to Serious Health Conditions," CDC.gov, May 26, 2020, https://www.cdc.gov/aging/publications/features/lonely-older-adults.html.

20. Jacob Ausubel, "Older People Are More Likely to Live Alone in the U.S. Than Elsewhere in the World, Pew Research Center, March 10, 2020, https://www.pewresearch.org/fact-tank/2020/03/10/older-people-are-more-likely-to-live-alone-in-the-u-s-than-elsewhere-in-the-world/.

21. Michael Toscano, "Continued Isolation will Kill More Elderly," The American Conservative, June 5, 2020, https://www.theamericanconservative.com/articles/continued-isolation-will-kill-more-elderly/.

22. Louise Aronson, "For Older People, Despair, as Well as Covid-19, Is Costing Lives," The New York Times, June 8, 2020, https://www.nytimes.com/2020/06/08/opinion/coronavirus-elderly-suicide.html?referringSource=articleShare.

23. Toscano, "Continued Isolation will Kill More Elderly."

24. "The COVID Pandemic Could Lead to 75,000 Additional Deaths from Alcohol and Drug Misuse and Suicide," The Well Being Trust, accessed January 8, 2021, https://wellbeingtrust.org/areas-of-focus/policy-and-advocacy/reports/projected-deaths-of-despair-during-covid-19/.

25. Olga Khazan, "The Millennial Mental-Health Crisis," The Atlantic, June 11, 2020, https://www.theatlantic.com/health/archive/2020/06/why-suicide-rates-among-millennials-are-rising/612943/.

26. Andrea Petersen, "The Toll That Isolation Takes on Kids during the Coronavirus Era," The Wall Street Journal, June 15, 2020, https://www.wsj.com/articles/the-toll-that-isolation-takes-on-kids-during-the-coronavirus-era-11592236617.

27. Petersen, "The Toll That Isolation Takes on Kids during the Coronavirus Era."

28. Petersen, "The Toll That Isolation Takes on Kids during the Coronavirus Era."

29. Elise Amez-Droz, "Caring for COVID-19 Patients and Staff in Nursing Homes," The Bridge, June 16, 2020, https://www.mercatus.org/bridge/commentary/caring-covid-19-patients-and-staff-nursing-homes.

30. Julia Marsh and Bernadette Hogan, "NYC, State Failed to Fund Nursing Home Watchdogs, Report Says," New York Post, June 17, 2020, https://nypost.com/2020/06/17/nyc-albany-failed-to-fund-nursing-home-watchdogs-report/.

31. Kristin Byrne, "'It Shouldn't Be Happening:' Elder Abuse, Neglect on the Rise in Milwaukee County during COVID-19," WTMJ-TV Milwaukee, June 17, 2020, https://www.tmj4.com/rebound/it-shouldnt-be-happening-elder-abuse-neglect-on-the-rise-in-milwaukee-county-during-covid-19.

32. Deborah Amos, "How the Pandemic Has Affected Patients in Hospice Care," National Public Radio, June 3, 2020, https://www.npr.org/transcripts/869053439.

33. Charlie Camosy, "Do We Do Everything in Our Power to Lower the COVID-19 Infection Rate?" Religion News Service, April 20, 2020, https://religionnews.com/2020/04/20/should-we-do-all-we-can-to-lower-the-

covid-19-infection-rate/.

34. Holbrook Mohr, Mitch Weiss, and Reese Dunklin, "Thousands Sick from COVID-19 in Homes for the Disabled, Associated Press, June 11, 2020, https://apnews.com/bdc1a68bcf73a79e0b6e96f7085ddd34?utm_campaign=SocialFlow&utm_medium=AP&utm_source=Twitter.

35. Joseph Shapiro, "COVID-19 Infections and Deaths Are Higher Among Those with Intellectual Disabilities," NPR, June 9, 2020, https://www.npr.org/2020/06/09/872401607/covid-19-infections-and-deaths-are-higher-among-those-with-intellectual-disabili.

36. Scott D. Landes et al., "COVID-19 Outcomes Among People with Intellectual and Developmental Disability in California: The Importance of Type of Residence and Skilled Nursing Care Needs," Disability and Health Journal, April 2021, https://www.sciencedirect.com/science/article/pii/S1936657420301898.

37. Pat Eaton-Robb and Susan Haigh, "Hospitals Ordered to Allow Support for Disabled Patients," Associated Press, June 9, 2020, https://apnews.com/9f93f9a3adcef9df1f77d138a0dc4963.

38. Quoted in Robb and Haigh, "Hospitals Ordered to Allow Support for Disabled Patients."

39. Christine Rousselle, "Burying a Loved One during a Pandemic," Washington Examiner, June 4, 2020, https://www.washingtonexaminer.com/opinion/burying-a-loved-one-during-a-pandemic?_amp=true&__twitter_impression=true.

40. Journal Staff, "Mass. Health Committee Makes History Approving End of Life Options Bill for First Time since 2011," Revere Journal, June 3, 2020, http://reverejournal.com/2020/06/03/mass-health-committee-makes-history-approving-end-of-life-options-bill-for-first-time-since-2011/.

41. Wesley J. Smith, "Dutch MD Euthanized Dementia Patient Despite Being Told 'No,'" National Review, June 15, 2020, https://www.nationalreview.com/corner/dutch-md-euthanized-dementia-patient-despite-being-told-no/.

42. "Doctor Cleared of Murder in Euthanasia Case Says She Would Do It Again," Dutch News.nl, June 15, 2020, https://www.dutchnews.nl/news/2020/06/doctor-cleared-of-murder-in-euthanasia-case-says-she-would-do-it-again/.

43. Smith, "Dutch MD Euthanized Dementia Patient Despite Being Told 'No'" (italics added).

44. Wesley J. Smith, "Assisted Suicide by Zoom," First Things, June 5, 2020, https://www.firstthings.com/web-exclusives/2020/06/assisted-suicide-by-zoom.

45. Haley Jena, "What a Pregnant ER Physician Wants You to Know about the Coronavirus," What to Expect, March 27, 2020, https://www.whattoexpect.com/news/family/leana-wen-pregnancy-coronavirus/.

46. Doug Dollemore, "The U Leads National Study of COVID-19 Effects on Pregnancy," The U, June 9, 2020, https://attheu.utah.edu/facultystaff/the-u-leads-national-study-of-covid-19-effects-on-pregnancy/.

47. Kyle Almond, "At Home or in the Hospital: Giving Birth during a Pandemic," CNN Health, accessed January 11, 2021, https://www.cnn.com/interactive/2020/05/health/coronavirus-pregnancy-birth-cnnphotos/index.html.

48. Good Morning America, "'Real Housewives' Star Kara Keough Bosworth Opens Up about the Heartbreaking Loss of Her Newborn Son," Facebook, May 11, 2020, https://www.facebook.com/GoodMorningAmerica/videos/2985785414823568/.

49. Oksana Grytsenko, "The Stranded Babies of Kyiv and the Women who Give Birth for Money," The Guardian, June 15, 2020, https://www.theguardian.com/world/2020/jun/15/the-stranded-babies-of-kyiv-and-the-women-who-give-birth-for-money.

50. Yuras Karmanau and Dmytro Vlasov, "Foreigners are Being Allowed into Ukraine to Collect Their Surrogate-Born Babies," TIME, June 10, 2020, https://time.com/5851739/ukraine-pandemic-coronavirus-surrogate-babies/.

51. Robert Winston and Rebecca Chicot, "The Importance of Early Bonding on the Long-term Mental Health and Resilience of Children," London Journal of Primary Care, February 24, 2016, https://dx.doi.org/10.1080%2F17571472.2015.1133012.

52. Alessandra Colaianni, "'For Now, We Wait': Postponing Cancer Surgery during the Coronavirus Crisis," The New Yorker, April 22, 2020, https://www.newyorker.com/science/medical-dispatch/for-now-we-wait-postponing-cancer-surgery-during-the-coronavirus-crisis.

53. Alex Hakim, "ICU Doctor: What I Wish People Knew about Coronavirus," The Federalist, May 8, 2020, https://thefederalist.com/2020/05/08/icu-doctor-what-i-wish-people-knew-about-coronavirus/.

54. William Saletan, "Abortion Funding Isn't as Popular as Democrats Think," Slate, June 12, 2019, https://slate.com/news-and-politics/2019/06/joe-biden-hyde-amendment-democratic-support.html.

55. Michael J. New, "New Poll Shows Small Gains in Pro-life Sentiment," National Review, June 12, 2020, https://www.nationalreview.com/corner/new-poll-shows-small-gains-in-pro-life-sentiment/.

56. New, "New Poll Shows Small Gains in Pro-life Sentiment."

57. New, "New Poll Shows Small Gains in Pro-life Sentiment."

58. Sarah McCammon, "Trump Administration to Planned Parenthood: Return Coronavirus Relief Funds," NPR, May 21, 2020, https://www.npr.org/2020/05/21/860410536/trump-administration-to-planned-parenthood-return-coronavirus-relief-funds.

59. Sen. Steve Daines et al. to Jovita Carranza, April 30, 2020, https://www.inhofe.senate.gov/imo/media/doc/4.30.20%20Daines-Rubio-Arrington-Johnson%20Letter%20to%20SBA%20Administrator%20re%20Planned%20Parenthood.pdf.

60. "Senate COVID-19 Response Package Leaves Much to Be Done for Our Families and Public Health Response," Planned Parenthood Action Fund, March 25, 2020, https://www.plannedparenthoodaction.org/pressroom/senate-covid-19-response-package-leaves-much-to-be-done-for-our-families-and-public-health-response.

61. Sen. Josh Hawley to Jovita Carranza, May 20, 2020, https://www.hawley.senate.gov/sites/default/files/2020-05/Hawley-Letter-SBA-Administrator-Planned-Parenthood-PPP.pdf.

62. Sarah McCammon, "Trump Administration to Planned Parenthood: Return Coronavirus Relief Funds," NPR, May 21, 2020, https://www.npr.org/2020/05/21/860410536/trump-administration-to-planned-parenthood-return-coronavirus-relief-funds.

63. Ted Budd and Marjorie Dannenfelser, "Abortion is Never Essential, Especially during a Pandemic," RHINO Times, April 23, 2020, https://www.rhinotimes.com/news/abortion-is-never-essential-especially-during-a-pandemic/.

64. David Lee, "Fifth Circuit Lets Texas Limit Abortions during Covid-19 Crisis," Courthouse News, April 20, 2020, https://www.courthousenews.com/fifth-circuit-rules-texas-can-restrict-medication-abortions-during-covid-19-crisis/.

65. Max Brantley, "8th Circuit Reinstates Arkansas's Ban on Surgical Abortions," Arkansas Times, April 22, 2020, https://arktimes.com/arkansas-blog/2020/04/22/8th-circuit-reinstates-arkansass-ban-on-surgical-abortions.

66. U.S. Court of Appeals for the Eighth Court, "In Re: Leslie Rutledge," no. 20-1701 (2020) https://ecf.ca8.uscourts.gov/opndir/20/04/201791P.pdf.

67. Carole Novielli, "The Abortion Pill: So Dangerous It Needs a Rare Safety Requirement," Live Action, June 6, 2020, https://www.liveaction.org/news/abortion-pill-dangerous-safety-requirement/.

68. Maarit Niinimaki et al., "Immediate Complications after Medical compared with Surgical Termination of Pregnancy," Obstetrics & Gynecology

114, no. 4 (2009): 795, https://doi.org/10.1097/aog.0b013e3181b5ccf9.

69. Kristi Stone Hamrick, "Abortion Pills Without Rh-Testing Could Prevent Many Women from Ever Having Children," Washington Examiner, May 29, 2020, https://www.washingtonexaminer.com/opinion/abortion-pills-without-rh-testing-could-prevent-many-women-from-ever-having-children.

70. Paul Strand, "Both Sides in the Abortion Battle See Changes Wrought by Coronavirus Pandemic," CBN News, May 14, 2020, https://www1.cbn.com/cbnnews/us/2020/may/both-sides-in-the-abortion-battle-see-changes-wrought-by-coronavirus-pandemic.

71. Denise Burke, "Pill Pushers Exploiting COVID-19 to Promote Risky Telemedicine Abortions," The Daily Signal, May 14, 2020, https://www.dailysignal.com/2020/05/14/pill-pushers-exploiting-covid-19-to-promote-risky-telemedicine-abortions/.

72. Michael Kunzelman, "Doctors Sue to Block FDA Abortion Pill Rule during Pandemic," ABC News, May 28, 2020, https://abcnews.go.com/Health/wireStory/doctors-sue-block-fda-abortion-pill-rule-pandemic-70927996.

73. Marjorie Dannenfelser et al. to FDA Commissioner Stephen Hahn, May 4, 2020, https://www.sba-list.org/wp-content/uploads/2020/05/AidAccess-Coalition-Letter-FINAL.pdf.

74. "'Unconscionable': Planned Parenthood Pres. Condemns States Using Pandemic to Limit Abortion Access," Democracy Now! April 27, 2020, https://www.democracynow.org/2020/4/27/coronavirus_us_abortion_access_texas_alabama.

75. Anna Reynolds, "Abortion Pill Reversal Hotline Receives Record Number of Calls during COVID-19," Pregnancy Help News, April 28, 2020, https://pregnancyhelpnews.com/abortion-pill-reversal-hotline-receives-record-number-of-calls-during-covid-19.

76. "Pills by Post—Abortion Pill Treatment at Home," British Pregnancy Advisory Service, accessed January 12, 2021, https://www.bpas.org/abortion-care/abortion-treatments/the-abortion-pill/remote-treatment/ (capitalization original).

77. Georgia Simcox, "Police Investigate Death of Unborn Baby after Woman Took 'Pills by Post' Abortion Drugs While 28 Weeks Pregnant—Four Past the Legal Limit," Daily Mail, May 23, 2020, https://www.dailymail.co.uk/news/article-8349739/Police-investigate-death-unborn-baby-woman-took-abortion-drugs-home-28-weeks-pregnant.html.

ARE YOU ETHICALLY PREPARED FOR THE NEXT PANDEMIC?

CHEYN ONARECKER, MD, MA

Introduction

Most of us have not faced the decimation caused by earthquakes, famines, hurricanes, tsunamis, and forest fires, but few of us have escaped the effects of the COVID-19 pandemic. The total numbers of infections and deaths worldwide are staggering—113,000,000 documented infections and over 2.5 million deaths as of February 2021.[1] Daily, we have watched the predictions change, wondering if our healthcare systems would be overrun by sick and dying patients, worried that our economies would not recover from the impact of the strategies employed to mitigate the effects of the disease. Over time it became clear that most of the hospitals in this country were not going to be overrun with COVID-19 patients. Although the devastation in the United States has been great—over 500,000 deaths[2]—we escaped the damage that was predicted in the early days of the pandemic. Experts at the Centers for Disease Control projected that as many as 200 million Americans would be infected and 1.7 million would die by the end of the summer of 2020.[3]

The truth is, we were caught off guard by COVID-19. We were not prepared for a public health crisis of this magnitude. We did not have enough beds or protective equipment or ventilators or space in the morgues. But we were not just unprepared from a medical logistics perspective. We were not prepared for the ethical challenges we were about to face either. As it looks now, we will not have to make the types of decisions that caused Italian physicians to weep in the hallways of the hospitals in Northern Italy. That gives us time. It gives us a chance to get ready. What did we learn from COVID-19 that will help us prepare for the next pandemic? Just as important as it will be to prepare ourselves medically for the next pandemic, we must be prepared ethically for the crisis that will inevitably come.

Given the magnitude of the task of planning for the medical and economic contingencies of another worldwide disaster like COVID-19, why should healthcare professionals spend our valuable time talking about the ethics of a pandemic? Because the decisions we will be forced to make in a public health crisis like a pandemic touch on some of the most deeply held convictions we have about what it means to be a healthcare professional. If we ignore the ethics, we will find ourselves working in an environment characterized by low morale and burnout, confusion about roles and responsibilities, mistrust among leaders and healthcare workers, and unjust treatment of vulnerable human beings. If we address these issues now, before the next crisis hits, and take the proper steps to prepare ourselves, we will experience increased morale and personal well-being, greater trust, more accurate and helpful communication, and the implementation of policies and protocols that guard the dignity of those who need our help the most.

We may have been unprepared, ethically, for the COVID-19 pandemic, but we must be ready for the next crisis. To prepare, we should focus on three ethics principles: the duty to treat, respect for the dignity of all persons, and caring for the caregiver.

The Duty to Treat

The first ethics question we need to answer is, what is a healthcare worker's duty to treat patients in a pandemic? In other words, do we have a responsibility to care for the sick when it puts our own health, or the health of someone we love, at risk? The words of an internal medicine resident at the University of California, San Francisco illustrate the struggle that all healthcare professionals experience as they balance the good of caring for sick patients with the risk to personal health:

> I find moral distress . . . in shuffling my delegated responsibilities . . . to my colleagues on the basis of fuzzy deductions. Plainly, I fear that an otherwise healthy colleague who covers my role could too acquire COVID-19 and suffer similar if not more severe consequences of the infection.
>
> In a time of pandemic and uncertainty, I wonder if I am shirking obligation. I fear caring for patients with COVID-19 because I fear my own risk . . . Yet do I have an obligation to patients to use my training to serve, despite fear and desire for distance? . . .
>
> Does a certain amount of public good outweigh risk in the medical field? How much risk in the career of medicine should be acceptable to physicians? I do not know that I will ever find the concrete answers to these questions.[4]

While it might be commendable for physicians to place themselves at risk during a public medical crisis, is it appropriate for society to expect them to do so? The AMA Code of Medical Ethics, for example, states: "Because of their commitment to care for the sick and injured, individual physicians have an obligation to provide urgent medical care during disasters. This obligation holds even in the face of greater than usual risks to physicians' own safety, health, or life."[5] Where does that obligation come from? Let me suggest four reasons.

First, we have greater skills and abilities to treat patients. A lifeguard on the beach has a greater obligation to rescue a drowning tourist than a bystander because he has had extensive training in water rescue. He has a greater ability to help. Second, because physicians have more medical training and expertise, they are better able to mitigate risks than someone who is not trained. They appreciate the importance of protective equipment and understand how to avoid spreading infections. Third, physicians have flourished because society grants us special privileges in exchange for the promise to help in crisis. We drive nice cars, wear nice clothes, and eat at nice restaurants, and society is OK with that. There is public support for healthcare education and training programs. Physicians and nurses are permitted to train on fellow human beings. We engage in procedures and high-risk interventions which other members of society are forbidden to do. And, perhaps most important of all, society allows us the autonomy to practice according to our own standards and to be our own police. In exchange for those benefits, the public expects that we will use our knowledge and skills to care for patients in need, even at risk of personal inconvenience, cost of time with family and friends, and risk of exposure to harm. No one forced us to become physicians. We volunteered.

And then there is a fourth reason—our calling. We have been called by God to serve our fellow human beings, those who bear the image of God. In the New Testament book of Philippians, Paul admonishes us to humble ourselves and demonstrate a greater concern for what matters to others instead of our own interests (Phil 2:3–4, NIV). John wrote that our love for others is the appropriate response to the love God first demonstrated to us (1 John 4:19). And Jesus himself said that he did not come to be served but to serve and to lay down his life for many (Matt 20:28). He said that the greatest commandment was to love God with all your heart, but he said there was a second commandment that ranked right up there with the first: love your neighbor as yourself (Matt

22:36–39). Throughout history, those who professed to be followers of Jesus cared for the sick and needy during epidemics. Even those who do not have a religious background were drawn to medicine by a deep conviction that their promise to care for their patients went far beyond a contract with an insurance company or healthcare organization. That conviction is what drew them in the first place and what sustains them during periods of great stress. We wanted a career in healthcare because we wanted to care for people. It is true for every physician and nurse I have ever met. And, the truth is, we expose ourselves to risk every time we care for a patient. There should be no question that physicians have a duty to treat patients in a pandemic.

But is that duty to treat absolute? In general, I think most of us would agree that as the risk of personal harm increases, the responsibility to provide treatment decreases. Where do we draw the line between actions that are simply part of our duty as healthcare professionals and actions that go way beyond the call of duty? Until the 1800s, over 2,200 years after Hippocrates, there had been no consistent professional tradition within medicine that expected physicians to care for patients when personal harm was at stake. For example, although he documented some of the signs and symptoms of soldiers suffering from the Antonine Plague, Galen did not risk his life to care for the sick and dying in second century Rome:

During the first plague, the famous classical physician Galen fled Rome for his country estate where he stayed until the danger subsided. But for those who could not flee, the typical response was to try to avoid any contact with the afflicted, since it was understood that the disease was contagious. Hence, when their first symptom appeared, victims often were thrown into the streets, where the dead and dying lay in piles.[6]

But in the first AMA Code of Ethics in 1847, a new professional obligation arose out of concern for the threats of impending epidemics. "When pestilence prevails, it is [the physicians'] duty to face the danger, and continue their labors for the alleviation of suffering, even at the jeopardy of their own lives."[7] The statement was unprecedented in the annals of the medical profession. And yet, in the history of medicine in this country over the past 175 years, it has been rare to find examples of physicians abandoning their patients in the face of personal risks.

What are the risks? According to the CDC, more than 400,000 healthcare workers in the United States have tested positive for COVID-19, and over 1,300 have died.[8] The risk is real, and it is more real for some of us than others. Patients with diabetes, COPD, chronic kidney disease, heart disease, obesity, and cancer, for example, have a higher risk of developing severe disease than those who are otherwise healthy. Those over the age of 50 are 10 to 15 times more likely to die from the disease than those in their 20s and 30s.[9] What is the level of risk beyond which we cannot expect our healthcare workers to practice? Should we hold our colleagues who are older, or those with chronic diseases, to the same expectations for seeing patients as those of us who are otherwise young and healthy? What about those, like me, who live with aged parents? Although my risk of severe disease is low, my exposure to COVID-19 patients could potentially endanger my mother's life.

And what about the lack of personal protective equipment (PPE)? Even now, over a year after the pandemic began, there is a shortage of N95 masks.[10] Whose obligation is it to take on the risk of exposure in the absence of proper PPE? If a police officer, firefighter, or soldier would not be deployed without proper protection, is it reasonable to ask a healthcare worker to face undeniable dangers without proper equipment? We must remember that the consequences of exposing healthcare workers to COVID-19 without adequate protection extends beyond the personal risk to the individual or family member. When physicians and nurses contract the disease, there are fewer workers to care for patients.

As physicians and nurses and hospital administrators wrestle with the most effective ways to deploy personnel and accommodate those who are at highest risk, they should base their decisions about a risk threshold on the healthcare worker's knowledge and skills, their personal health, and balancing the benefits of treating patients with the risks of exposure and the loss of resources should the worker become ill. Keep in mind that the duty to treat may be fulfilled in ways other than in-person care. Healthcare workers can conduct virtual visits, facilitate accurate and up-to-date communication between leaders and caregivers, and educate and support those who provide direct patient care.

I believe we have a duty to treat. We are better trained, we have the knowledge and skills to reduce personal risks, we have a promise to keep to the ones who have supported our decisions to pursue careers in medicine, and our service is the fulfillment of our desire to become healthcare professionals and the only appropriate response to God who loved us and called us to serve. The bottom line is there is no established formula or guideline for determining in all situations the level or degree of risk that distinguishes an extravagant act from the ordinary act of doing what duty requires. The threshold will be different for each person, and to be effective in caring for patients in a public health crisis, we must determine what our responsibility is.

Respect for Persons

Once we clarify our duty to treat patients during the pandemic, we must develop plans to allocate resources should our systems become overwhelmed. A pandemic creates a situation in which the usual standards of medical treatment come under severe stress. Resources are strained and there is great pressure to lose the focus on the importance of the individual. We must be careful, as we adjust to the lack of adequate equipment, supplies, and personnel, to not be carried away by a strictly utilitarian strategy. The protocols we design must be grounded in the foundational concept that every human being is created in the image of God and has inestimable intrinsic worth and dignity.

As we have seen during the COVID-19 crisis, we can adjust to accommodate a surge of patients by increasing the production of critical supplies and equipment, optimizing the supplies and medical treatments that we have, creating additional space in our hospitals, building new facilities, and moving ventilators to where they are needed most. But, in a true crisis situation, when resources are exhausted, the approach of "business as usual," or the delivery of care on a first-come, first-served basis, driven by the clinical judgment of physicians for individual patients, no longer holds. Instead, government and healthcare leaders will focus on "the greatest good for the greatest number," where "good" is defined by lives saved, life-years saved, or some similar outcome. The goal in these situations is sufficient care, also referred to as *crisis standards of care*, rather than the normal standard of care. In other words, policies will emphasize rendering the best possible medical care, but given the limited resources, the level of care will be less than what patients receive under non-crisis situations.

This shift in the overall approach to patient care cuts to the core of our calling as healthcare professionals. Edmond Pellegrino said that "the first principle of medical ethics, the end to which it is directed, is the good of the patient."[11] Since the days of Hippocrates, our charge, as physicians, has been to work for the benefit of the individual who is asking us for help. In a public health crisis, when the demand for care exceeds our resources, no longer is the individual the only consideration. Instead of saving one patient, we are being told to save as many lives as possible. Unless you have been in an emergency room during a mass casualty event or involved in battlefield medicine, you will not be prepared for this shift. The change in priorities is a painful one and can create significant moral tension and even moral distress for everyone involved.

To resist the impulse to adopt a completely utilitarian focus, we must hold on to the values that first brought us in to medicine. We cannot let society's emphasis on "the greatest good for the greatest number" trample our respect for the intrinsic value of all human beings. Decisions must be equitable and based on objective and justifiable medical criteria as well as informed clinical judgment. Crisis standards of care must be non-discriminatory and not based on perceived social worth, ethnicity, age, gender, sexual orientation, religious convictions, disability, or any other medically non-relevant trait that does not impact crisis-related prognosis. Upholding the belief in the intrinsic value of all human beings will help healthcare professionals navigate through the controversies that arise when trying to create acceptable triage protocols.

What are the most common controversies? First, should certain groups be excluded from treatment? For example, some protocols discriminate against patients with severe chronic conditions like end-stage renal disease, class III or IV heart failure, and dementia by excluding them from ICU care altogether, without clear justification. Those chronic conditions that affect prognosis should be included in the calculation, but they should not be used to exclude patients from care. Some protocols set an age cutoff. Douglas White and Bernard Lo explain, however, that such exclusions imply that those patients' lives are not worth saving, which could lead to outright discrimination. Also, the exclusions are not practically useful in a surge crisis, because available equipment and medications will surge and decline episodically during the pandemic.

Finally, they point out that the policy violates a fundamental principle of public health ethics: use the means that are least restrictive to individual liberty to accomplish the public health goal.[12]

Second, should healthcare workers and first responders be given priority? Advocates of this position appeal to the principles of reciprocity and instrumental value to justify such a conclusion. Reciprocity refers to the reward that healthcare workers should get in exchange for being willing to put themselves at risk. Knowing that you will be one of the first to receive critical care might encourage you to be a part of the front lines rather than retreating to the shadows. Instrumental value means that society will benefit from restoring healthcare workers to health as quickly as possible to get them back to caring for patients. In the case of COVID-19, though, how realistic is it to think that a person requiring intensive care services will soon be in any condition to get back to caring for patients? In specific circumstances, such as the allocation of vaccines, a policy that favors healthcare workers might be acceptable, but in most cases, there is no reason to prefer healthcare workers over others.

Third, should ventilators and medications be allocated solely based on who is most likely to survive to hospital discharge? White and Lo consider that, by itself, this is an ethically insufficient justification. In their view, it is also relevant to consider the number of life years saved by calculating what is called near-term survival.[13] In other words, it would be better to provide a ventilator to someone who is likely to live for another 40 years than a person who is likely to die within four years. The difficulty with such a calculation is that a simple number cannot determine which of two lives is more valuable. First, it is impossible to know for certain that the one individual will live for 40 years. And it may be that the other individual will make more of their four years than the one will make of their 40. Second, using near-term survival to allocate ventilators and medical treatments is likely to discriminate against the disabled who already live with many chronic and debilitating illnesses. Better to restrict survival calculations to determine those who are most likely to survive the immediate acute illness and prevent unequal treatment of the disabled. At the very least, if some sort of near-term calculation is included, then only those conditions that have reached terminal stages should be considered.

Fourth, should young people have priority over the aged? Many ethicists recommend that younger persons should receive priority, not because they are worth more to society than older persons, but because they have not had a chance to live through life's stages. This consideration is referred to as the life-cycle principle. It seems to me, however, that using life cycles as a criterion is a subtle way of discriminating against the elderly. And which life events should receive priority? For example, during a crisis, who should get the ventilator: a 45-year-old with a family of five, or a 35-year-old who is single? Are we really supposed to prioritize the 35-year-old?

Fifth, what about the disabled? People without disabilities, including medical providers, tend to rate the quality of disabled persons' lives far lower than disabled people rate their own quality of life.[14] Triage protocols have included factors such as chronic disabilities in their determination of short-term prognosis. But disabled people, who already feel that their lives are undervalued, fear that they will be undertreated and less likely to receive life-sustaining treatment. In an article entitled "Will They Take My Vent?" "Alice Wong, a disability activist and PV [personal ventilator] user, explains this concern: 'Were I to contract coronavirus, I imagine a doctor might read my chart, look at me, and think I'm a waste of their efforts and precious resources that never should have been in shortage to begin with. He might even take my ventilator for other patients who have a better shot at survival than me."[15]

Sixth, what about ethnic minorities? African Americans and Hispanics are becoming infected with COVID-19 and dying at a higher rate than white Americans. Multiple factors contribute to the increased numbers including higher burdens of comorbid disease, poverty, poor health care access, infeasibility of social distancing due to living in densely-populated neighborhoods and households, and the need to continue to work in public-facing occupations.[16] How do we overcome the disadvantages suffered by these communities? Most of the issues that affect these outcomes occur long before the patient arrives in the emergency department. Some advocate preferentially allocating resources to men and women of color to overcome the disadvantages that they have had in accessing the healthcare system and benefitting from the resources that most of us take for granted by using a weighted lottery system.[17] While this might not adhere to the principle of maximizing the greatest good for the greatest number, advocates say it would be a helpful step to restore faith in the government and healthcare institutions for a large number of Americans. Others point out, however, that we do not have an equitable way of determining which patients' medical conditions have been the most affected by social and economic disadvantages.

With these controversies in mind, what principles can guide us to develop fair triage protocols? This is not an exhaustive list, but I believe these seven guidelines will ensure that our protocols uphold the dignity of all persons.[18]

1. Triage and allocation decisions should be prioritized, primarily, based on medical need and likelihood of surviving the acute illness. The concept of near-term survival can also be employed, but with caution. Although important, placing too great a prior-

ity on any parameter other than surviving the acute illness may further disadvantage those who already have significant disabilities.

2. Fairness requires triage and resource allocation to pay particular attention to the needs of at-risk and marginalized persons, including the poor, the aged, minorities, and persons with disabilities. That means that triage protocols should be developed with input from representatives of these communities. Also, institutions can train triage teams and oversight committees on avoiding discrimination.

3. Criteria (e.g., age, chronic diseases, disabilities) that exclude patients from access to critical services under any circumstances should not be used.

4. If resources are available, they should be deployed as indicated. Decision tools should not be used to exclude patients preemptively from use of life-saving resources when these resources are available.

5. Even during a surge crisis, the treating physician or healthcare worker has a paramount duty to care for the individual patient. Triage and resource allocation decisions that apply to individual patients should be the responsibility of parties other than the treating physician. This is best accomplished through a triage officer or team who is removed from direct patient care and work in close partnership with a facility's ethics committee.

6. Patients who have deteriorated and are no longer eligible for life-saving resources (e.g., mechanical ventilation) are never to be abandoned and should continue to receive intensive symptom management as well as psychosocial and spiritual support. Where available, palliative care teams should be involved.

7. Physicians should have a formalized procedure to advocate for

their patients regarding individual triage decisions, including an expedited appeal process.

What about the special situation of reallocation? What is reallocation? In a crisis surge situation, reallocation is withdrawing life support, without the agreement of a surrogate or the directions of an advance directive, with the direct intent of transferring that same life-supportive treatment to another patient who has been deemed more worthy of the device. Imagine that you have only one ventilator. Patient A has been on the ventilator for 24 hours and, although the patient has not deteriorated, she is not improving as quickly as we hoped, and it is not clear that she will make it. Patient B arrives and has a better short-term survival prognosis. Reallocation would require that the ventilator be withdrawn from Patient A and given to Patient B. The justification is that the scarce resource, the ventilator, would be used most efficiently, because Patient B has a better prognosis. However, it is well known that the clinical course for COVID-19 patients waxes and wanes. While Patient A's status may be worse today, she is not imminently dying, and she may improve. Withdrawing the ventilator from Patient A guarantees her death. Unless Patient A is imminently dying, it would be unethical to remove her ventilator to treat Patient B. Not only would it be unethical, it may also be illegal. What if the family of patient A refuses to let us stop the ventilator? Non-consensual withdrawal of life-support is extremely controversial. Even in Texas, where the Advance Directive Act allows unilateral withdrawal of life support in special situations, the law is being challenged.[19]

Are there steps we can take to help us avoid a situation where reallocation is even a consideration? Yes. First, hospitals and community leaders must create triage protocols that match patients with the resources they need. Second, physicians should not offer treatments that will not benefit patients, even when requested by a surrogate. Third, when talking about ventilators with patients and families, physicians should present such treatments as a time-limited trial to set appropriate expectations. The time-limited trial must be long enough to avoid removing ventilators from patients who would have survived with a little more time. Otherwise, with ventilators starting and stopping so often the ICU could look like a game of musical chairs. Fourth, the triage team or officer should make these decisions. The treating physician is going to be trying hard to save his patient and does not need the extra conflict of making that decision. Fifth, hospitals must institute palliative care in all cases where life support is discontinued and arrange for family members to be present.[20]

Finally, governments and institutions have an ethical obligation to plan allocation of critical scarce resources through a process that is transparent, open, and publicly debated to the extent time permits. All triage operations should be regularly and repeatedly evaluated to guarantee that the process has been followed fairly, that the need for triage operations still exists, that current criteria continue to be based on the best available evidence, and that the dignity of human beings continues to be respected even in the midst of the frenzy.

Caring for the Caregivers

We have spent some time looking at two important ethics principles that bear directly on how we, as healthcare professionals, should direct our efforts during a pandemic. First, we know we have a duty to treat, even in the face of personal risk. Second, we realize the need to develop policies in an open, transparent way that upholds the dignity of all persons. Now let us turn to the ethical responsibility of institutions and society toward healthcare workers. Think of this as caring for the caregivers.

Healthcare professionals on the front lines of the pandemic cannot win this battle alone. Medical institutions and society also have duties to healthcare workers who place themselves in harm's way in the care of patients. Based on my clinical experience during COVID-19 and the literature already cited, the three duties are to: 1) provide protection for healthcare workers to the extent that protection is possible, 2) furnish healthcare workers with the tools necessary to treat the sick, and 3) provide appropriate care for healthcare workers suffering from burnout, moral distress, and other mental health disorders. Institutional leaders should remember that individuals are more likely to be committed to serving their institution, even to the point of going beyond the call of duty, when they feel there is unswerving commitment from the institution in which they serve.

First, institutions must protect their workers. Other first responders are not expected to risk their lives without proper protective equipment, so we should not expect healthcare workers to routinely care for infected patients without protection. Almost a year after the pandemic began, clinics and hospitals faced a shortage of N95 masks. In an article entitled, "Somehow, We Still Don't Have Enough N95 Masks," Susan Bailey, president of the American Medical Association said, "Physicians, nurses, and other frontline providers risk their lives every day to take care of COVID patients, and they're being asked to do things that they would have been disciplined for doing prior to the pandemic."[21]

Second, clinicians need to have the tools to test and treat patients. Despite assurances from government leaders that testing supplies were adequate, when the second wave of the pandemic hit in the fall, local hospital labs were overwhelmed, diagnostic testing centers were constantly behind, and turnaround times increased significantly.[22] Longer turnaround times affect decisions regarding treatment, the length of quarantine periods, and contact tracing, and increase the risk that healthy persons may be exposed. Even more frustrating has been the lack of effective treatments. Beneficial effects of the vaccine are months away, so proven therapies are vital to prevent death and disability from the disease. Currently available medications, however, have shown only limited success.

Third, we must care for the emotional needs of the caregiver. Healthcare workers on the front line are at risk of developing moral distress, burnout, and other mental health symptoms. In a survey in January 2020 of 1,257 healthcare workers in China, 61% were nurses and 39% were physicians. 76% of the participants were women, and 65% were between the ages of 26 and 40. 50% of those taking the survey reported symptoms of depression, 45% reported anxiety, 34% suffered from insomnia, and 71% reported psychological distress.[23] In Italy, half of front-line healthcare workers experienced symptoms of post-traumatic stress disorder. Almost 25 percent of workers suffered from depression and roughly 20 percent reported symptoms of anxiety.[24]

A study of 1,119 U.S. healthcare workers caring for COVID-19 patients was conducted in 2020 by Mental Health America. Eighty-two percent reported emotional exhaustion, 70% had trouble with sleep, 68% were physically exhausted, and 63% dreaded work. Over half experienced loss of appetite, chronic headaches, or abdominal pain. More than three quarters of healthcare workers with children said they were worried about exposing their child to COVID-19, nearly half of responders were worried about exposing their spouse or partner, and 47% were worried that they would expose their older adult family members. Fifty-five percent were considering a change in career.[25]

Healthcare workers feel isolated from family and friends and exhausted by long hours. For nurses, routine duties are just piled on to the extra time that it takes to care for COVID-19 patients. When one of their colleagues is sick or quarantined, the rest of the team works the extra hours to cover the gap. The medical staff follow detailed steps for getting in and out of their protective equipment, knowing that a misstep makes them vulnerable to infection. Every day the thought goes through their minds: Is today the day I make a mistake and carry the infection home to my family? As a result, many are afraid to touch their husbands or wives or children after work. They skip out on holidays and other important celebrations to protect their family and friends from possible infection.

Physicians and nurses speak about the sadness of holding the hands of patients as they die. Since family members are rarely present in the intensive care units, the staff become their families. One hospitalist said to me, "We have plenty of ventilators, but not enough nurses and physicians to manage them." She had seen more death in the previous three weeks than she had in the previous ten years. The worst part of her job was making the phone call to inform the family that their loved one had died. Over the past few months, she said, she had made far too many phone calls, and rarely did a day go by that did not end in tears.[26]

When physicians are forced to make decisions in a public health crisis that would not have been made in normal circumstances, they risk suffering from moral distress and injury. A patient who might have lived two weeks ago is now receiving comfort care because of a lack of ventilators. A patient who would benefit from antiviral medications may not make it because the remaining doses were used on another patient. Physicians can begin to experience intense feelings of shame, guilt, or disgust which can lead to depression, post-traumatic stress disorder, and suicidal ideation.[27]

For many reasons, healthcare workers may not request support if they are experiencing stress reactions. So, employers should be proactive in encouraging supportive care and take the following steps.[28]

1. Provide good quality communication and accurate informational updates to all staff. At my hospital throughout the pandemic, we have had Skype and Zoom meetings, it seems, around the clock. But those meetings have been crucial in helping us make sense out of what is going on around us and finding ways to work together to solve some of the enormous challenges we were facing. The communication must be two-way, open to staff input and concerns.

2. Incorporate mental health risk reduction strategies in the workplace. Create work breaks and adjust schedules; regularly rotate workers out of high stress tasks; prevent isolation and facilitate social interaction; and establish regular check-ins with colleagues, family, and friends. Assign tasks to teams and create an environment of patience and hope. Encourage the institution's mental health professionals to meet regularly with the staff and consider establishing support groups such as Schwartz Rounds.[29]

3. Educate staff on where and how they can access mental health and psychosocial support services and make it easy for them to use the services.

4. Train each member of the healthcare team to recognize the signs of depression and assist affected team members to find help.

Conclusion

A pandemic like COVID-19 can overwhelm our healthcare systems and force us into crisis standards of care that challenge the very nature of what it means to be a healthcare professional. As healthcare leaders and institutions reflect on the strengths and weaknesses of our response to COVID-19, no doubt many of us will be part of strategic planning teams to make sure we are prepared, medically, for the next crisis. But we must also be prepared ethically. By focusing on the three key ethics principles discussed in this paper we will build trust, increase morale, decrease misinformation, and protect the dignity of our patients. We have a duty to treat, before God and our fellow human beings, even in the face of personal risk. We must uphold respect for the dignity of all persons, even amid depleted resources. And we must care for the health-care workers who are on the frontlines of the crisis.

Endnotes

1. WHO: WHO Coronavirus Disease (COVID-19) Dashboard, February 28, 2021, https://covid19.who.int/.

2. Centers for Disease Control and Prevention, "COVID Data Tracker: Global Counts and Rates," CDC.gov, updated February 28, 2021, https://covid.cdc.gov/covid-data-tracker/#global-counts-rates.

3. Sheri Fink, "Worst-Case Estimates for U.S. Coronavirus Deaths," New York Times, March 13, 2020, https://www.nytimes.com/2020/03/13/us/coronavirus-deaths-estimate.html.

4. Cynthia Tsai, "Personal Risk and Societal Obligation Amidst COVID-19," JAMA 323, no. 16 (2020): 1555–56, https://www.doi.org/10.1001/jama.2020.5450.

5. American Medical Association (AMA), "Physicians' Responsibilities in Disaster Response & Preparedness: Code of Medical Ethics Opinion 8.3," November 14, 2016, https://www.ama-assn.org/delivering-care/ethics/physicians-responsibilities-disaster-response-preparedness.

6. Rodney Stark, The Triumph of Christianity: How the Jesus Movement Became the World's Largest Religion (New York: Harper One, 2011), 114–15.

7. AMA, Code of Medical Ethics of the American Medical Association (Chicago: AMA Press, 1847), 105.

8. Centers for Disease Control and Prevention, "COVID Data Tracker: Cases & Deaths among Healthcare Personnel," CDC.gov, updated February 28, 2021, https://covid.cdc.gov/covid-data-tracker/#health-care-personnel.

9. Centers for Disease Control and Prevention, "Risk for COVID-19 Infection, Hospitalization, and Death by Age Group," CDC.gov, updated February 18, 2021, https://www.cdc.gov/coronavirus/2019-ncov/covid-data/investigations-discovery/hospitalization-death-by-age.html.

10. Adele Peters, "Somehow, We Still Don't Have Enough N95 Masks," Fast Company, December 18, 2020, https://www.fastcompany.com/90587753/somehow-we-still-dont-have-enough-n95-masks.

11. Edmund D. Pellegrino, The Philosophy of Medicine Reborn: A Pellegrino Reader, ed. H. Tristram Engelhardt and Fabrice Jotterand (Notre Dame, IN: University of Notre Dame Press, 2008).

12. White and Lo, "A Framework for Rationing Ventilators and Critical Care Beds During the COVID-19 Pandemic," 1773.

13. White and Lo, "A Framework for Rationing Ventilators and Critical Care Beds During the COVID-19 Pandemic," 1773.

14. Mary Crossley, "Ending-Life Decisions: Some Disability Perspectives," Georgia State University Law Review 33, no. 4 (2017): 900–901, https://

readingroom.law.gsu.edu/cgi/viewcontent.cgi?article=2897&context=g-sulr.

15. Laura Guidry-Grimes and Katie Savin, "'Will They Take My Vent?': Ethical Considerations with Personal Ventilator Reallocation During COVID-19," Bioethics.Net, April 15, 2020, http://www.bioethics.net/2020/04/will-they-take-my-vent-ethical-considerations-with-personal-ventilator-reallocation-during-covid-19/.

16. CDC, "Coronavirus Disease 2019 (Covid-19): Health Equity Considerations and Racial and Ethnic Minority Groups," July 24, 2020, https://www.cdc.gov/coronavirus/2019-ncov/need-extra-precautions/racial-ethnic-minorities.html.

17. Douglas B. White et al., "Model Hospital Policy for Fair Allocation of Scarce Medications to Treat COVID-19," University of Pittsburgh Department of Critical Care Medicine, May 28, 2020, https://ccm.pitt.edu/sites/default/files/2020-05-28b%20Model%20hospital%20policy%20for%20allocating%20scarce%20COVID%20meds.pdf

18. Paul Hoehner et al., "Triage and Resource Allocation during Crisis Medical Surge Conditions (Pandemics and Mass Casualty Situations): A Position Statement of the Christian Medical and Dental Associations Special Task Force, Christian Journal for Global Health 7, no. 1 (2020): 45–55, https://journal.cjgh.org/index.php/cjgh/article/view/387/735.

19. Bethany Blankley, "U.S. Supreme Court Rejects Hospital's Attempt to End Baby Tinslee's Life," The Center Square, January 20, 2021, https://www.thecentersquare.com/texas/u-s-supreme-court-rejects-hospital-s-attempt-to-end-baby-tinslee-s-life/article_db586262-5b55-11eb-b8b4-177cb12dbb86.html.

20. White and Lo, "A Framework for Rationing Ventilators and Critical Care Beds During the COVID-19 Pandemic," 1774.

21. Peters, "Somehow, We Still Don't Have Enough N95 Masks."

22. Ken Alltucker, "The Demand for COVID-19 Testing Is Up, Stressing Labs and Delaying Results," USA Today, November 26, 2020, https://www.usatoday.com/story/news/health/2020/11/26/covid-19-testing-delays-record-demand-thanksgiving/6417506002/.

23. Jianbo Lai et al., "Factors Associated with Mental Health Outcomes among Health Care Workers Exposed to Coronavirus Disease 2019," JAMA Network Open 3, no. 3 (2020): e203976, https://www.doi.org/10.1001/jamanetworkopen.2020.3976.

24. Rodolfo Rossi et al., "Mental Health Outcomes among Frontline and Second-Line Health Care Workers during the Coronavirus Disease 2019 (COVID-19) Pandemic in Italy," JAMA Network Open 3, no. 5 (2020): e2010185, https://www.doi.org/10.1001/jamanetworkopen.2020.10185.

25. Mental Health America, "The Mental Health of Healthcare Workers in COVID-19," MHAnational.org, https://mhanational.org/mental-health-healthcare-workers-covid-19 (accessed January 6, 2021)

26. Personal communication with author.

27. Neal Greenberg et al., "Managing Mental Health Challenges Faced by Healthcare Workers during Covid-19 Pandemic. BMJ 368:m1211 (2020): https://www.doi.org/10.1136/bmj.m1211.

28. National Center for PTSD, "Managing Healthcare Workers' Stress Associated with the COVID-19 Virus Outbreak," U.S. Department of Veterans Affairs, March 2020, https://www.ptsd.va.gov/covid/COVID19Managing-StressHCW032020.pdf.

29. The Schwartz Center for Compassionate Healthcare, "Schwartz Rounds and Membership," theschwartzcenter.org, https://www.theschwartzcen-ter.org/programs/schwartz-rounds/ (accessed August 30, 2020).

CONTRIBUTORS

Matthew Lee Anderson is a Postdoctoral Research Fellow at Baylor University's Institute for Studies of Religion and an Associate Fellow of the McDonald Centre for Christian Ethics. His academic work is focused on articulating the grounds for procreative and parental rights and countering anti-natalist arguments. He founded *Mere Orthodoxy*, an online journal devoted to faith, culture, and politics, and is the author of *Earthen Vessels* and *The End of our Exploring*. He is a Perpetual Member of Biola University's Torrey Honors Institute.

F. Matthew Eppinette is Executive Director of The Center for Bioethics & Human Dignity (CBHD). He holds a PhD in Theology from Fuller Theological Seminary. He is a graduate of the MA Bioethics program at Trinity International University, and has an MBA from Louisiana Tech University. He previously served as New Media Manager and Executive Director of the Center for Bioethics and Culture, where he co-wrote and co-produced six documentary films addressing bioethics issues. Dr. Eppinette's current research interests include transhumanism, Alasdair MacIntyre's ethics and epistemology, and the intersection of fiction, film, and other areas of culture, particularly popular culture, that raise or address bioethics issues.

Catherine Glenn Foster serves as President & CEO of Americans United for Life. She earned her JD at Georgetown University Law Center and also holds an MA in French from the University of South Florida. Foster has authored and testified on numerous domestic, foreign, and international legislation and initiatives, as well as white papers, articles, and op-eds. She has testified before and advised the U.S. Senate Judiciary Committee, the U.S. House of Representatives Committee on Energy and Commerce Select Investigative Panel and Subcommittee on Oversight and Investigations, and other federal and state bodies and representatives.

Wilson Jeremiah is a faculty member at Southeast Asia Bible Seminary (SEABS), Malang, East Java, Indonesia. He receives his MDiv in Theological Studies from his beloved alma mater (SEABS), and his ThM in Philosophical and Moral Theology from Calvin Theological Seminary. He is currently pursuing a PhD in Systematic Theology at Trinity Evangelical Divinity School, where he was the recipient of the 2020–2021 Robert D. Orr Endowed Fellowship and served as the managing editor for *Dignitas* and *Intersections* for The Center of Bioethics and Human Dignity.

Bryan Just serves as Event & Executive Services Manager at The Center for Bioethics & Human Dignity (CBHD). He graduated with a BA in Psychology from Nyack College and MAs in Theological Studies and Church History from Trinity Evangelical Divinity School. His master's thesis covers the history of CBHD and its place in Evangelical bioethics.

Dónal O'Mathúna's interests focus on evidence-based practice and bioethics, with recent work on disasters and humanitarian crises. He has co-edited three volumes: *Ethics and Law for Chemical, Biological, Radiological, Nuclear & Explosive Crises* (2019), *Disasters: Core Concepts and Ethical Issues* (2018), and *Disaster Bioethics: Normative Issues When Nothing is Normal* (2014). He is particularly interested in the ethics of research in humanitarian crises. He has led funded research projects in this area, contributed to ethics initiatives and guidelines with the World Health Organization, UNICEF and the UN agency for disaster risk reduction (UNISDR), and published widely, including in *Lancet* and *Bioethics*.

Cheyn Onarecker is the director of St. Anthony Family Medicine Residency in Oklahoma City, Oklahoma. After completing a family medicine residency and a fellowship in academic medicine, he and two colleagues started the St. Anthony program with a mission *"to develop competent and compassionate family physicians who reveal the healing presence of God through exceptional healthcare and Christ-like character."* He is a member of the St. Anthony Hospital Ethics Committee and has been serving on the hospital triage team during the Covid-19 pandemic. Dr. Onarecker is also an adjunct professor in bioethics at Trinity International University.

Simiyu Bramwel Wekesa is a dedicated medical officer of health and a holder of Master of Arts in Bioethics from Trinity International University, Chicago. He is currently in his third year in of residency in Family Medicine and Community Health in Kabarak University, Kenya. His training site for the residency is AIC Kijabe Hospital. He is passionate about ethics in clinical practice of medicine and formulation and adherence to proper policies and laws in medical practice.

Joseph Wiinikka-Lydon is a researcher and lecturer at a European Union-funded Center for Ethics outside of Prague. Trained in religious and philosophical ethics, he writes on issues of moral injury, war and peace, and violence and subjectivity. His latest work is *Moral Injury and the Promise of Virtue*, published with Palgrave MacMillan.